"*Taking Charge of Your Own H...* ...umers trying to find their way through the maze of our health-care system. By relating her own amazing journey and those of others, Ms. Hall enlightens consumers on what health-care providers already know: Patients, together with supportive family members, are their own best advocates when seeking high-quality, safe care."

—MAUREEN CONNOR, RN, MPH
Former Vice President for Quality Improvement and Risk Management
Dana-Farber Cancer Institute, Boston, MA

"Lisa Hall's *Taking Charge of Your Own Health* is full of wisdom gathered from her own nine-year struggle to regain wellness, as well as being a thorough survey of the less-than-perfect U.S. health-care system. Follow her lead: Become informed, ask questions, consider the many options available to you, and become an active partner in your own health-and-wellness team!"

—SCOTT PARAZYNSKI, MD
Former NASA Astronaut and Mount Everest summiteer

"Lisa Hall has thoroughly investigated every facet of health care to provide tools and tips that are useful to anyone seeking solutions to medical problems…*Taking Charge of Your Own Health* provides an insider's guide to acquiring the best medical care possible."

—JAMES CONWAY
Senior Vice President, Institute for Healthcare Improvement

TAKING CHARGE
OF YOUR OWN HEALTH

LISA HALL
with Ronald M. Wyatt, MD, MHA

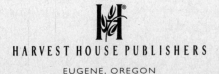

HARVEST HOUSE PUBLISHERS

EUGENE, OREGON

Cover by Dugan Design Group, Bloomington, Minnesota

Cover photos © ShulteProductions / iStockphoto; James Steidl / Fotolia; author photo on back cover by Blue Sky Photography, Madison, AL, www.blue-sky-photography.com

This book is not intended to take the place of sound professional medical advice. Neither the author nor the publisher assumes any liability for possible adverse consequences as a result of the information contained herein.

The names and details of some individuals whose circumstances are mentioned herein have been altered to protect their privacy.

TAKING CHARGE OF YOUR OWN HEALTH
Copyright © 2009 by Lisa Hall
Published by Harvest House Publishers
Eugene, Oregon 97402
www.harvesthousepublishers.com

Library of Congress Cataloging-in-Publication Data
    Hall, Lisa, 1962-
    Taking charge of your own health / Lisa Hall, with Ronald Wyatt.
    p. cm.
    ISBN 978-0-7369-2479-5 (pbk.)
    1. Self-care, Health. I. Wyatt, Ronald. II. Title.
    RA776.95.H355 2009
    613—dc22

                       2009017194

To my beloved mother, Patricia K. Hall.

Mom was the epitome of quiet strength and dignity even in the face of adversity. Without fail, she put others first, right up until her last hours on earth. We never had to earn her love or support; it was always unconditional.

Thanks, Mom. This is for you.

Contents

Part 1: Taking Responsibility for Your Health

Part 2: Taking Charge of Your Attitude

Quick-Reference Guide
to Information Sections

Foreword

Congratulations! You have just taken a very important step toward optimal health. Knowledge is power, and *Taking Charge of Your Own Health* will empower you to get the most out of your medical care.

Author Lisa Hall has thoroughly investigated every facet of health care to provide tools and tips that are useful to anyone seeking solutions to medical problems. Her passion for quality patient care was born of the frustrations she experienced during seven years of misdiagnosis and nine years of disability. She understands the challenges faced by people dealing with medical adversity because she has experienced them firsthand.

Ms. Hall enlisted the help of internal-medicine specialist Ronald Wyatt, MD, MHA—who is also a fellow of the Institute for Healthcare Improvement—to gather information for this comprehensive resource. Dr. Wyatt offers the perspective of a 20-year healthcare veteran and the passion of a physician who entered the profession for all the right reasons. He stops at nothing to find the correct diagnosis and treatment for all of his patients. He views his profession as an art as well as a science.

Taking Charge of Your Own Health provides an insider's guide to acquiring the best medical care possible. You will learn how to select the right medical practitioner, which safety guidelines are most critical in a hospital setting, and what to do when you need emergency care. You will discover strategies for disease prevention and early detection; preparing for doctor visits; searching the plethora of online medical resources; appealing an unpaid insurance claim; and finding free or reduced-cost drugs and medical, dental, and optical care.

This comprehensive resource includes input from physicians, nurses, patients, the Joint Commission, the Institute for Healthcare Improvement, the American College of Surgeons, and many others. Ms. Hall solicited input from physicians nationwide through an online survey on such topics as elusive diagnoses, patient responsibilities, critical screenings, hospital errors, managed care, and how they choose their own physicians.

Patient Empowerment

In the seminal publication issued by the Institute of Medicine (IOM) in 2001, *Crossing the Quality Chasm,* ten new rules were given to guide patient, doctor, and nurse relationships, including supporting the patient as the source of control. According to the IOM, patients should be given the necessary information and the opportunity to exercise the degree of control they choose over health-care decisions that affect them. The IOM also noted that the health-care system should be able to accommodate differences in patient preferences and encourage shared decision-making.

Patient empowerment has become more critical than ever, with shortages of internists and family-practice physicians as well as the increased pressure on clinicians to see more patients per day—leading to shorter office and hospital visits and far more responsibility for self-management of one's health.

However, the news is very exciting when consumers engage. National and international projects are demonstrating exceptional results when patients are given and assume responsibility for their own care. *Taking Charge of Your Own Health* gives you the tools and knowledge to assume this responsibility proactively and confidently. Good luck and good health!

JAMES CONWAY
Senior Vice President
Institute for Healthcare Improvement

A Partnership Effort

How many times have you sought help from your doctor, expecting an immediate diagnosis and treatment, only to hear, "The test results are negative. There's nothing wrong with you." Or even worse, the doctor says, "I know exactly what it is! Take this medication, and you'll feel much better." When you try the medication, nothing happens and your troubling symptoms remain.

Unfortunately, medicine is not an exact science. That's not to say that physicians don't deserve the utmost respect for selecting a difficult career that typically requires seven years of postgraduate education. They have chosen a challenging profession that often presents elusive cases and limitations imposed by our health-care system. The medical field is fraught with diagnostic, surgical, and medication errors; mismanaged hospitals; insufficient emergency care; and inadequate patient insurance coverage. These pitfalls necessitate a partnership between doctor and patient for checks and balances. And, yes, it has to be a partnership, as both depend heavily on one another to arrive at the correct diagnosis and treatment.

Physicians have the scientific training and the analytical skills needed to find the proper diagnosis and treatment. However, they cannot feel the symptoms and the impact they have on the patient's life. They must depend on patients to describe the severity, frequency, and impact of their symptoms clearly. Diagnosis and treatment must be a collaborative effort between doctor and patient.

Physicians depend on patients to do some of the investigative work. Even the most dedicated doctor does not have the time or passion that a desperate patient or loved one has to search for answers. A good case

in point is the story told in the book *Lorenzo's Oil*. Lorenzo's parents
worked tirelessly to discover a new treatment for the devastating disease adrenoleukodystrophy,* from which their son suffered. Because of
their efforts, Lorenzo's oil has shown preventive effects in patients with
X-linked adrenoleukodystrophy (Siva 2005).†

I realized the significance of doctor-patient collaboration during my
own amazing medical journey. My primary care physician, Dr. Ronald
Wyatt, was the cornerstone of my care and a huge source of support. He
ruled out a number of conditions and referred me to specialists until the
thirty-eighth physician ultimately diagnosed and treated my debilitating
condition. I eagerly sought Dr. Wyatt's help in developing content for
this book. His insight and expertise allowed me to get inside the mind
of a physician while writing from a patient's point of view.

Taking Charge of Your Own Health started out as a memoir of my own
experiences and lessons learned along the way that can benefit others. With
Dr. Wyatt's guidance, it has evolved into a how-to guide for any patient
seeking diagnosis, treatment, and even illness prevention. Throughout
this project, I have interviewed over 70 medical and legal professionals
and patients to gather information on topics such as misdiagnosis, hospital
safety, medication safety, wellness and preventive medicine, emergency
medical care, alternative care, insurance dispute resolution, disability and
workers' compensation guidelines, and pain management.

Misdiagnosis is one of the biggest challenges faced by both physicians
and patients. According to Medical Malpractice Lawyers and Attorneys
Online, approximately 40 percent of all medical malpractice claims are
filed because of failure to diagnose a medical condition in a timely manner. Additional surveys suggest that up to 40 percent of all diagnoses
may be wrong (Oz 2006, 232). Watch any episode of *Mystery Diagnosis*

---

* For definitions of this and other medical terms, see the "Guide to Medical Terminology" starting
  on page 225.

† Throughout this book I have used the author-date system of notes. A brief description of the source
  appears in parentheses after the citation, and full source information is given in the references in
  the back of the book.

on the Discovery Health Channel, and you will see the devastation an undiagnosed or misdiagnosed condition has on a patient's life.

My story would have ended much differently if I had given up after doctor number three or doctor number twenty-two or even doctor number thirty-seven. I had decided early in my journey that if I could keep persevering, there was at least a chance I could turn this difficult situation around. If I gave up and did nothing, the situation was nearly guaranteed to remain unchanged. Additionally, the action of perseverance was so empowering that I did not feel victimized by my circumstances. I took charge of my life and my health.

Now I am on a new mission—to empower you with what I have learned and to provide practical applications to help you take charge of your own medical care. I learned techniques like creating spreadsheets for my current medications, all attempted treatments, chronic conditions, past surgeries, and past hospitalizations. I created a system for collecting and organizing my medical records so physicians could scan the material quickly. I am eager to share these and other tools and techniques, along with the knowledge I amassed during my long search for answers.

My story is testimony to the human spirit and to the strength that lies deep within each of us. God gives all of us a deep reserve of strength. He blesses some of us more than others with opportunities to test that strength, but He never gives us more than we can handle. On several occasions, when I thought I was at my breaking point and could not go on, and when all doors seemed closed, a glimmer of hope would appear. During nine years of disability, while I was unable to drive a car or live a normal life, God never abandoned me. This experience strengthened my faith as I sought to understand why God chose this journey for me. As I write this book, I now understand.

Into the Abyss

My Search for Diagnosis

The hospital has just released you from a five-day stay. "You're on the mend. You should feel much better in a week," the doctor says. You eagerly envision getting back to your busy life. Everything is fine—you think.

On the way home, you stop at the drugstore with your spouse to fill prescriptions. But suddenly, you realize something is terribly wrong. As you get out of the car, you can't walk more than five feet without becoming dizzy and disoriented. Everything is so dark and tilted, and there are flashes like strobe lights. You feel as though you're walking on pillows. You're disconnected from your body, and your legs don't obey your brain when you try to walk. You notice a strange hissing sound in your ears.

When you get home, the situation isn't any better, and you find it difficult to navigate around the house. When you try to drive your car, it feels as though you are floating through outer space. You can't feel your hands on the steering wheel or your foot on the gas and brake pedals. You did not have any of these symptoms prior to your hospitalization. *It's the residual effects of the hospitalization,* you decide. *They're just temporary.*

Little do you know this is just the beginning of a nearly decade-long nightmare.

This nightmare has dominated my life since February 1995. Prior to the onset of the mystery condition, I lived a full and happy life. I worked full time as a human-resources administrator at a large aerospace company in Huntsville, Alabama. My husband, Joe (pseudonym), and I shared our home with two beautiful German shepherds, Brandy and Sheba. Life was good, and the future looked very bright.

My entire world collapsed on February 22, 1995. I had begun to feel ill the previous evening, and then I vomited throughout the night until I finally lost consciousness. My fever rose to 104 degrees, the abdominal pain was horrendous, and the pain in my knees rendered me nearly unable to walk. I had a severe headache and was very weak. Joe was out of town on a business trip. He had just started working for a new company and was at the corporate headquarters a thousand miles away for new-employee orientation. I was scared to death to be in this condition by myself.

I knew that I was in trouble because I had experienced these symptoms in 1990, and my fever then had gone up to 105 degrees. The doctors had finally diagnosed my symptoms in 1991 as ulcerative colitis, a form of inflammatory bowel disease and a chronic disease of the colon, or large intestine, marked by an abnormal response from the body's immune system. Typical symptoms include abdominal cramping, bloody diarrhea, nausea, vomiting, and fever. Nonintestinal symptoms can include joint pain, skin lesions, and even eye irritation. The symptoms of ulcerative colitis tend to come and go, with periods of remission in between flare-ups. My 1990 episode had been undiagnosed and untreated, and I later found out it could have been fatal had I not been otherwise young and healthy. When I recognized these same symptoms in 1995, I knew I needed to get to the emergency room. I held on until a reasonable hour of the morning to call for help from my neighbor, and she quickly drove me to the hospital.

The emergency department physician called my primary-care physician (PCP) and my gastroenterologist. They believed that I was suffering from a severe flare-up of ulcerative colitis, brought on by a new antibiotic and they all agreed to admit me. The doctors gave me intravenous fluids and Solu-Cortef, a steroid drug. I didn't like the idea of the steroid's side effects, but my gastroenterologist said it was the only way to save my colon. My neighbor called Joe, gathered my things for me, and took care of Brandy and Sheba. I was relieved that everything was under control at home and very grateful for her help.

Throughout my five-day hospital stay, I was on a clear-liquid diet of broth, Jell-O, juice, Popsicles, and soft drinks. Joe came home the day after my admittance, still in shock at the turn of events. He visited me daily, bringing balloons and a card on my thirty-third birthday. He offered to bring in a birthday cake, but my strict diet did not allow that. He picked me up on my last day in the hospital, thankful that things were getting back to normal. I was looking forward to going home, resting for a week or so, and then getting back to work and my busy life.

I left the hospital in a wheelchair, as hospitals always require, and got into the car. Joe and I stopped at a small drugstore to get my prescription filled. That was when I first noticed the bizarre symptoms I had not had prior to hospitalization. It was difficult to walk even a few feet in the store because I felt disconnected to my feet. I felt as though there was a short circuit between my brain and feet. *Why is walking so difficult? And why does everything appear so dark?* I sensed flashing, and everything I looked at was tilted to the right. Although I could hear people's voices, they sounded muddled and far away. And then I noticed a constant, strange hissing sound—like loud snow on a television. I had to find a bench to sit down on while Joe got my prescriptions.

During the next few days, I rested a lot. Everything seemed so difficult and took ten times more effort than before. I tired easily and stayed disoriented pretty much all the time. The hissing in my ears drove me crazy, and then I noticed a new symptom, a weird ammonia-type odor. I smelled it in every room of the house and outside. Nobody else could detect it. *What is going on?* I wondered, and I started to panic because these symptoms were new and seemed to have nothing to do with ulcerative colitis.

Nearly a week passed after my release from the hospital. I planned to return to work the next day and decided the weird symptoms were just going to have to wait, go away, or something. Symptoms or no symptoms, I had a career and an employer who needed me. The night before I returned to work, Joe and I walked next door to thank our neighbor for her help. During that short walk, I felt as though I was not going to make it. I was dizzy, disoriented, and unable to make my feet connect with the ground. Throughout our visit, I felt disoriented, and the room spun and swam. I felt like Dorothy in *The Wizard of Oz* before the tornado. *What's tomorrow going to bring if tonight is this bad? I have to get back to work,* I thought when I got home.

I'll never forget the commute to work the next day. I started the car, pulled out of the driveway, and turned from our street onto the main road. But something didn't feel right. Everything looked darker than it should, surreal, dreamlike. The car was floating along, and I didn't feel connected to it. I didn't feel as though my hands were on the steering wheel or my foot was on the gas or brake pedal. The passing scenery seemed to swim before my eyes. *This will stop,* I kept thinking. *Soon I'll feel like I'm driving.*

If I hadn't been in total denial about what was happening and how bad it was, I would've pulled over and called for help. But I kept thinking, *This isn't happening—it isn't supposed to be happening! The doctor said I could go back to work in a week, and the week's up.*

Somehow I made it to work, and everyone was glad to see me back but concerned about what I'd experienced. It was evident that I had lost eleven pounds in a week, which might have made me happy under better circumstances. I felt totally disoriented as I walked down the hall to the break room to get something to drink, and I couldn't make it all the way back to my office. I had to stop in the restroom and lie down for a while. We had a midmorning staff meeting, and things really started spinning and swimming when everyone began talking at once. I had to get up and leave. In the privacy of my office, I burst into tears and called Joe to come and get me. We left my car at the office, and weeks passed before I attempted to drive again.

The next day, Joe took me to see the gastroenterologist, who suspected the steroid medication was causing side effects that could explain these mysterious symptoms. He also said that I would have to continue the oral steroid drug Prednisone for four months to get the ulcerative colitis completely under control. *I'll never be able to stand these bizarre symptoms for four months! I'll never make it!* I thought. I had no idea what kind of nightmare awaited me. I didn't know this was the end of life as I had known it.

The debilitating symptoms persisted for another nine long years. During this time, I could not work, drive a car, or walk more than 20 or 30 feet. On one occasion, I got stranded at the end of my driveway because my brain could not process the passing scenery and it disoriented me; a neighbor helped me back into the house. I started using a cane and sometimes a wheelchair. I could not shop in most stores because of my brain's inability to tolerate stimuli such as sights, sounds, and fluorescent lighting. The most frustrating part was not knowing what it was, how to fix it, or how to explain my deficits to others. I was beyond mortified when I had to try and explain to someone why I couldn't walk into a grocery store and needed a wheelchair. I can't begin to describe the self-loathing that accompanied this very dark period.

During the next seven years, I consulted 37 medical practitioners in a desperate attempt to get my life back. Joe and I traveled to the Mayo Clinic, Johns Hopkins University Hospital, the University of Alabama Hospital in Birmingham, the Shea Ear Clinic, and Vanderbilt University Hospital. We also consulted doctors in Virginia, Tennessee, Pennsylvania, and Florida. I eventually hired drivers to help with my many doctor visits in Huntsville and specialist consultations in Birmingham. I covered just about every medical specialty possible: internal medicine; neurology; neuropsychiatry; neuropsychology; opthaneurology; ear, nose, and throat; endocrinology; rehabilitation; chiropractic; and various areas of alternative medicine.

Unflattering Labels

Throughout my search for answers, I was diagnosed with everything from "organic mood disorder" to "suffering from conflict about her role as a Southern woman" and "depression" (who wouldn't be depressed?) to "obsessive-compulsive disorder." A neuropsychologist conducted a battery of tests, including IQ. When the result was much lower than previous IQ tests, she suggested that the earlier tests were not standardized and concluded that I was probably not that smart to begin with!

I endured nearly 40 different medical tests, and doctors looked at my brain, heart, autonomic nervous system, vestibular system, proprioceptive system, optical system, adrenal glands, hormones, pituitary gland, and mental health. Several doctors recommended psychiatric testing when they couldn't find the real problem, and this led to some bizarre experiences. One psychiatrist presented me with a large stack of pictures of ugly, unsmiling people and instructed me to pick out the ones I liked best, second-best, third-best, and the least. I told him I didn't like any of the pictures; they were all ugly. He pressured me, and I finally made some random selections. The results supposedly suggested a tendency toward manic depression, a diagnosis I had not heard before or since this goofy test.

In 1997, I was in a state of desperation and using a wheelchair, and I consulted a neuropsychiatrist. He ordered a PET (positron emission tomography) scan of my brain and found abnormalities in both temporal lobes. His diagnosis was temporal lobe epilepsy. He also reviewed my history and made a connection that no other doctor had found. He believed that the high fever or the steroid medication I'd had in the hospital in 1995 was the trigger after 18 years of cumulative trauma to my central nervous system. The trauma had been caused by the 105-degree fever in 1990, two concussions earlier in life, and a lightning injury when I was a teenager. (I'd been hit by lightning through an open window and thrown 12 feet into the next room.)

Joe and I were initially encouraged by this new diagnosis because it was backed by an abnormal PET scan. The neuropsychiatrist recommended various anticonvulsants, and I tried nine in all. None of them helped, and some of them made the symptoms worse. This doctor recommended more radical tests and treatments, including a test that involved drilling holes into the skull and putting electrodes on the brain—while I was awake. I said, "No, thank you." When he recommended medical morphine and heroin, I decided it was time to look in another direction.

The most painful procedure I endured throughout this entire nightmare was a 48-hour, video-monitored EEG (electroencephalogram), an inpatient procedure. To look at my temporal lobes, the neurologist implanted a three-inch wire into the side of my face. The nurse numbed my face first, but I still felt the wire in my gums, and it hurt so badly that my blood pressure plummeted and I nearly fainted. A patient in the next room did faint during this same procedure. Unfortunately, the test came back negative.

Most of the tests were negative, and each negative result was more devastating than the last. To make matters worse, a number of doctors delivered the news with comments like, "Good news. There's nothing wrong with you!" or, "You're lucky there's nothing seriously wrong with you." I don't think these doctors intended to trivialize my situation; they just didn't get it. I became so frustrated that I envied people with multiple sclerosis and curable forms of cancer. At least they knew what they were facing.

Early in my journey, I was blessed with a wonderful ally in my fight for an accurate diagnosis and treatment. In 1996, I consulted Dr. Ronald Wyatt. God was clearly watching out for me. I could not have found a better primary care physician for my complicated case. Dr. Wyatt referred me to a number of specialists, and he encouraged my Internet research and was not threatened by it. But most important, he believed in me and never once doubted that I had a legitimate, debilitating medical condition. He knew there was a problem, and he wanted to fix it nearly as badly as I did. Without his support, I never would have survived this ordeal.

Dr. Wyatt found the first clue that there was indeed a physical problem and it was not "all in my head." In 1996, he discovered that my blood pressure dropped by 16 points when I stood up quickly, indicating orthostatic hypotension, a sudden fall in blood pressure that occurs upon standing upright. He prescribed the drug Florinef to help regulate my blood pressure, but my symptoms did not improve.

During the next several years, other tests provided hints of something wrong but did not pinpoint the problem. The positive PET scan in 1997 had indicated abnormalities in both temporal lobes of the brain; an MRI (magnetic resonance imaging) spectroscopy in 1997 showed three possible abnormalities in the brain; thermography tests in 1998 and 2001 suggested problems with the autonomic nervous system; an eye-tracking test in 1999 showed severe deficiencies that indicated a problem in the brain; and testing by an occupational therapist in 2000 suggested sensory integration dysfunction. Unfortunately, none of these tests provided the answer to my biggest question: *How can I get my life back?*

In an effort to determine what role, if any, the lightning injury played in my condition, I joined Lightning Strike and Electric Shock Survivors, International in 1998. I found out through this group that lightning and electric shock injuries can cause symptoms that appear years later, and I met several people who had some overlapping symptoms, although none of them had an identical list of symptoms.

Throughout the years, doctors recommended various medications and treatment options, some based on test results and others on symptoms. There were 41 in all, ranging from anticonvulsants to antidepressants and antipsychotics to antihistamines and various rehabilitation exercises. Two treatments helped slightly and temporarily: photonic stimulation and power yoga. Photonic stimulation was an experimental treatment at the time, administered by an alternative practitioner in Pittsburgh, Pennsylvania. After a series of treatments, I felt slightly better for three or four months. I did not improve enough to drive a car or get my life back, but I was able to tolerate stimuli a little bit better. The yoga helped me improve from a 30-percent functioning level to about 50 percent. I now believe the yoga was helpful because I was in an inverted position when I was doing it, and this increased my blood pressure. After a year and a half, my body seemed to become acclimated to the yoga, and I regressed to about 30 percent of normal. This was the lowest point in my journey, because I had absolutely no hope and no prospects.

In spring 2001, I mentioned my frustrations to a neighbor, who recommended an ear specialist, Dr. Dennis Pappas in Birmingham, Alabama, 100 miles from my home. Dr. Pappas clearly respected me and took me seriously; I had found another important ally who played a pivotal role in helping me get my life back. He conducted a battery of inner-ear tests and definitively ruled out vestibular problems. He said he felt the problem involved brain function and recommended that I get a tilt-table test at the University of Alabama at Birmingham Hospital.

This test measures the autonomic nervous system's responses and uncovers abnormalities in it.

Although I had already had a tilt-table test with inconclusive results, Dr. Pappas felt it was worth another look. He explained that Dr. Cecil Coghlan, a cardiologist at UAB, was one of the country's foremost experts in the interpretation of tilt-table tests. The downside would be a six-month wait for the report from this high-demand doctor.

During the test, the technician indicated the appearance of possible abnormalities, and I was encouraged. A positive test result may be bad news for some, but for anyone desperately seeking a diagnosis, it is the best news possible. However, while I waited six months for the test results, I continued looking for answers elsewhere.

Six months later, Dr. Pappas's office contacted me and scheduled a consultation to discuss my tilt-table test results. Sure enough, the report showed glaring abnormalities that indicated an autonomic nervous system dysfunction. I was afraid to even hope that this was a good sign. By this time, I was totally beaten down by my circumstances and reluctant to be even cautiously optimistic. Dr. Pappas recommended that I see Dr. Phillip Watkins, a cardiologist and medical director of the Autonomic Nervous Disorders and Mitral Valve Prolapse Center of Alabama.

Two months later, in February 2002, I met Dr. Watkins, my third powerful ally. He concurred that the test showed abnormalities that could cause all of my symptoms. I was skeptical because I had heard similar comments from other doctors before. He asked if I had ever taken Zoloft, a serotonin reuptake inhibitor, and I said that I had. He then asked if I had tried Florinef, and I said I had. When he asked if I had tried them together, I said no. He suggested that we play chemist and find the right combination of medications to increase blood flow to the brain. He recommended the Zoloft-Florinef combination, but he cautioned that it might take several trials to find the magic formula.

Despite my skepticism, I agreed to give it a try. As I was leaving, he sent me to the lab on the next floor for blood work. By this time, I was so disoriented from the stimuli of the previous four hours that I could not walk into the lab even with a cane and with my driver, Linda, leading me around. When we got off the elevator in the lobby, things were spinning and swimming so badly that I collapsed on the floor. I was in bad shape and desperately hoping, as I had many times before, that this treatment was the answer.

Four weeks later, with Linda's help and the use of my cane, I was able to walk into a department store and stay long enough to try on several dresses. I had not been able to do this before starting the Zoloft-Florinef combination. Linda and I cautiously discussed the possibility that I might be improving. Could this new regimen possibly be the answer to my prayers, after all these years?

The Doctor's View
Ronald Wyatt, MD, MHA

Lisa Hall was referred to me by a local specialist. She had a constellation of symptoms, including tinnitus, visual-spatial disturbance, dizziness and vertigo, vision changes, and balance problems. She walked with the use of a cane, and she could not drive or even walk very far with her beloved pets, Brandy and Sheba. Her past history was most pertinent for ulcerative colitis, and she told me that her symptoms seemed to have been caused by a recent flare-up that was accompanied by fever. She had been treated with high-dose steroids and probably had some degree of adrenal insufficiency from tapering off the steroid medication too rapidly.

After reviewing her history and symptoms, I felt it best to first develop a differential diagnosis, excluding common disorders first. Testing included basic metabolic parameters, thyroid function, the adrenal axis, and cardiac function. The initial evaluation did not reveal much, but I was very impressed with her story despite the paucity of objective findings. Ms. Hall seemed very reliable and much focused on finding out what was wrong and how to fix the problem.

She always kept her appointments and documented her symptoms and observations meticulously. I was impressed that she was very engaged in finding out what was wrong and that she was very goal-oriented. An important part of her clinical evaluation included a psychiatric evaluation, by me. Although she was anxious, I did not find any reason to think that she had a major psychiatric disorder. Her anxiety was appropriate for a formerly high-achieving professional who was now barely able to function independently.

I am certain that there were times she probably wondered if I thought she was mentally unstable, but I just never got that impression. She was encouraged to continue keeping observational notes of her symptoms and what she experienced in different settings when exposed to a variety of stimuli. I realized that some of her symptoms were postural, meaning they occurred when she assumed or was in an upright position.

The next phase of her evaluation looked for more esoteric problems. This list included disorders such as acoustic neuroma and other brain tumors; brain aneurysm, or what is called an A-V malformation in the brain, which would shunt venous blood and arterial blood in the wrong direction; pituitary gland tumor; atrial myxoma (heart tumor); autonomic nervous system dysfunction; atypical seizures or even pseudo-seizures; slow virus; demyelinating brain disease such as MS; and carcinoid syndrome. On a subsequent office visit, I found that she indeed had significant symptomatic orthostatic hypotension (low blood pressure), which was a big clue to the origin of some of her symptoms.

Ms. Hall later underwent a tilt-table test at the University of Alabama Birmingham's Kirklin Clinic. Cecil Coghlan, MD, world-renowned in the field of autonomic dysfunction, evaluated Ms. Hall's test results and concluded that she had autonomic nervous system dysfunction. However, while many of her symptoms were attributable to this disorder, I remained skeptical that it was the singular cause of all of her symptoms and findings.

My personal struggle was with the idea referred to as Occam's razor, which means that, all things being equal, the simplest solution is best. In internal medicine, one of the goals is to exclude all factors and elements that have nothing to do with the presumed diagnosis and to be able to attribute significant and objective findings to one or as few diagnoses as possible. In other words, why give a patient three or four diagnoses when one diagnosis can explain the entire process or, more succinctly, give a common cause of all symptoms.

Ms. Hall was very relieved by this confirmation from objective testing that it was not "all in her head," as other health-care providers had implied. She consulted Dr. Phillip Watkins, director of the Autonomic Disorders and Mitral Valve Prolapse Center of Alabama, who prescribed a treatment regimen that completely changed the course of Ms. Hall's life. As she made gradual but significant improvement, we began to search for the underlying cause of the autonomic dysfunction. We considered the numerous factors she shares in her story. Was it the lightning injury, the concussions, the high fevers, the steroid medication, or a combination? And what role did the positive PET scan play in her condition? Did damage to the brain cause the autonomic disorder, or did the autonomic disorder cause a section of the brain to appear damaged in the scan? And why was a subsequent scan performed at a different imaging center read as normal by a different specialist?

We may never have all the answers, but what we do know is that Ms. Hall has regained her life through sheer determination, intuition, and a healthy dose of obstinacy. On numerous occasions, I entered the exam room to find her seething after yet another specialist had failed to find the correct diagnosis but had recommended one more psychiatric evaluation. Her anger seemed to fuel her determination to prove the "blame-the-patient" brigade wrong. Had she deferred to the doctors who told her it was "all in her head," she would still be walking with a cane, unable to drive a car, and unable to live a normal life.

My listening skills, observational skills, and ability to empathize were all tested with almost every one of Ms. Hall's office visits. Gradually I saw her gaining knowledge and insight, and I watched her desire to find the cause of her malady evolve into a spirit of determination I had never encountered before. She decided early on not to allow herself to surrender to the impressions of many good physicians, acquaintances, and friends. We both reviewed the information and knowledge she gained from each medical encounter. We worked as a team to avoid duplication of services and to follow up on even the most subtle abnormalities in lab tests and other diagnostic evaluations as we attempted to make the correct diagnosis and formulate a management plan.

Ms. Hall's disorder not only tested my clinical skills, but it reminded me of why I chose this profession and specifically internal medicine as a career. Her journey has been a tremendous learning process for me.

I write this not only to help you understand Ms. Hall's condition from a practitioner's point of view, but also to encourage you in your own search for good health care. Ms. Hall made me a better listener, even though I had thought I was a good listener to begin with. I was motivated to read more on her symptomatology and to work harder as a medical detective to piece together the clues in an effort to unify her diagnosis.

If you take a similar attitude in your interaction with health-care professionals, you also will be able to find those practitioners whom you can motivate and inspire to do their best. In Ms. Hall's case, we now have a management plan that includes a team of providers, with Ms. Hall serving as equal partner in the process. This book she has written shows you how to reach a similar place in your journey. After all, it is your good health that is at stake.

Part I:

Taking Responsibility
for Your Health

Chapter 1

"Treatment Is 95 Percent Diagnosis"

How to Help Your Doctor Find a Correct Answer

An astute neurologist once told me, "Treatment is 95 percent diagnosis." In other words, a patient has just a 5 percent chance of stumbling upon a recovery without the correct diagnosis. The obvious solution is to get the correct diagnosis, but, as you can see, it is not that simple. My search for an accurate diagnosis took seven years, and others have suffered even longer.

The Problem of Misdiagnosis

In *How Doctors Think*, author Dr. Jerome Groopman cites the case of a young woman who suffered from severe gastrointestinal symptoms over a 15-year period. She became violently ill whenever she tried to eat, and the problem worsened progressively throughout the years. She consulted nearly 30 doctors and was diagnosed incorrectly with anorexia nervosa and bulimia. Her weight plummeted to 82 pounds, and she was severely malnourished. She was advised to eat 3000 calories per day and to include large quantities of bread and pasta. Did any of these doctors look at a correlation between her bread and pasta consumption and her symptoms and think to test for celiac disease? Not for 15 years. A gastroenterologist finally solved the mystery and undoubtedly saved this patient's life (Groopman 2007, 1-3).

Horror stories of no diagnosis, delayed diagnosis, and misdiagnosis abound within the health-care industry, with an estimated misdiagnosis rate of 40 percent. Nancy suffered with a diseased gall bladder for three long years before receiving a correct diagnosis, despite textbook symptoms of nausea, vomiting, and pain below the sternum and in the upper back. She found relief only after visits to six different doctors. Kathie suffered with connective tissue disease for five years and visited a dozen different doctors before Dr. Wyatt correctly diagnosed and treated her condition. Karen Grove, creator of the Grove Approach, a program to lessen the effects of fibromyalgia, suffered with the disease for six years before receiving the proper diagnosis.

Gall-bladder disease, connective-tissue disorders, and fibromyalgia are all fairly common yet commonly misdiagnosed. How can people with rare conditions expect to receive an accurate diagnosis? In a cruel twist of irony, Kathie's daughter, Kristina, became critically ill while Kathie was adjusting to life with her own chronic illness. Kristina suffered from severe abdominal pain and vomiting that caused her weight to drop to 80 pounds. She found partial relief after she had surgery to remove her gall bladder, but her stubborn symptoms continued despite a number of diagnostic tests that showed normal results.

Fortunately, Kristina's employer was a compassionate primary-care physician, who tirelessly sent her to a number of specialists. A gastroenterologist finally looked at her extensive history and previous tests and, using the process of elimination, determined that the condition had to be Sphincter of Oddi, a very rare, debilitating condition. Kristina had corrective surgery, and her symptoms disappeared. But throughout their journeys, Nancy, Kathie, Karen, and Kristina all heard at least one practitioner say that their conditions were "all in their head" or of psychological origins.

The Consequences

Misdiagnosis and delayed diagnosis have broad ramifications. At the very least, they cause prolonged, unnecessary suffering. In many cases, the lack of a documented diagnosis makes it impossible for patients to qualify for disability through a private insurer, Social Security disability, or workers' compensation. Prolonged symptoms of unknown origin, or "unknown etiology" in doctor-speak, can also cause the erosion of interpersonal relationships, including marriage. The undiagnosed patient is often perceived as a malingerer.

Because of misdiagnosis, doctors administer the wrong medication for the wrong condition, which is not only expensive, but dangerous. Linda consulted a rheumatologist for severe joint pain and was mistakenly diagnosed with ankylosing spondylitis. The rheumatologist prescribed the powerful drug Methotrexate via injection. This drug is known to cause severe or even life-threatening side effects. As it turned out, Linda's joint pain was the result of ulcerative colitis, and she realized that the Methotrexate was unnecessary only after receiving several doses of it.

The psychological effects of misdiagnosis can be nearly as bad as the symptoms themselves. Laurie Todd found herself on an emotional roller coaster while fighting for her life and trying to figure out what she was fighting, all at the same time. When she began to suffer from fatigue and a swollen abdomen, she scheduled a physical exam with a doctor in her HMO and was declared "the healthiest 55-year-old on the planet." Three months later, she sought another opinion, and a CT (computed tomography) scan revealed that she probably had stage III or IV ovarian cancer. After surgery, she received the good news via phone that the mass was benign and she did not have cancer. A week later, Laurie's surgeon informed her that she had indeed had cancer, a nonaggressive appendix cancer called pseudomyxoma peritonei. He told her it had a 30 percent chance of recurrence during the next five years and recommended watchful waiting.

When Laurie carefully researched pseudomyxoma peritonei online, she found that this type of cancer is deadly when untreated. Armed with the information she had found in the *Annals of Surgical Oncology* and the *European Journal of Oncology*, she consulted an in-network oncologist, who told her that her cancer was rare and not much was known about it. He told her that she had "about two good years left" and said that the HMO doctors would repeatedly drain fluid from her abdomen as the cancer recurred. Had Laurie followed his protocol, she would not have lived to fight for the out-of-network treatment that saved her life, a battle that inspired her to write her book, *Fight Your Health Insurer and Win: Secrets of the Insurance Warrior*.

The most serious consequence of misdiagnosis or delayed diagnosis is death. The gravity of this problem is evident in the book *What You Don't*

Know Can Kill You: A Physician's Radical Guide to Conquering the Obstacles to Excellent Medical Care by Dr. Laura Nathanson. Dr. Nathanson lost her beloved husband, Chuck, to a rare tumor of the thymus. Upon investigation, she found that his peach-sized tumor had shown up in an X-ray but had gone undetected by at least six doctors for 22 months. His condition would have been curable had he been diagnosed correctly at the first appearance of the tumor (Nathanson 2007). My own mother fought a similar battle, and I tell her story at the end of this chapter.

The Survey

Misdiagnosis is such a source of frustration for both patient and physician that I felt compelled to explore this topic from a physician's perspective. In addition to vital input from Dr. Wyatt, I also gathered information from physicians in a variety of disciplines using a nationwide survey. Many of the survey questions, which you can read on my Web site, www.theproactivepatient.com, specifically address misdiagnosis, and the answers offer insight into the challenges faced by physicians.

One of the survey questions asks physicians for the number-one cause of misdiagnosis: 48 percent answered, "inadequate patient history"; 20 percent answered, "premature diagnosis"; 20 percent answered, "limitations imposed by managed care"; and 12 percent answered, "other." The most common "other" causes included poor-quality imaging, lack of communication between patient and physician, pre-existing prejudices and limitations in thinking by both patient and physician, rarity of disease, patients' dishonesty, and patients' resistance to psychiatric or chronic medical diagnosis.

Given the many obstacles, how does a physician arrive at a correct diagnosis? Although patients look to physicians for answers, the answers are often complex and elusive. With thousands of identified diseases that may present differently from one patient to another, physicians must weigh a number of factors when seeking the correct diagnosis and treatment (Improving Diagnostic Accuracy 2007, 1).

An astute diagnostician considers the set of symptoms and looks first at the most common diagnosis that would explain the symptoms. Because of the time spent on common diagnoses, more esoteric diagnoses are more difficult. Many physicians employ a maxim known as Occam's razor, which recommends the removal of all unnecessary assumptions and pursuit of the simplest solution.

The diagnostic process starts with the all-important patient history. One survey respondent emphatically stated, "The patient *always* tells you where the problem is." The Physician Survey (see sidebar) results show a significant reliance on patient history. When asked how many elusive cases physicians diagnose through patient histories rather than X-rays or labs, 33 percent of respondents answered, "50 to 60 percent"; 22 percent responded, "30 to 50 percent"; 18 percent answered, "65 to 80 percent"; 15 percent answered, "0 to 35 percent"; and 12 percent responded, "over 80 percent."

After careful review of the patient's medical history, a good clinician performs an extensive review of each body system, followed by a complete physical exam. After completing this process, she develops a differential diagnosis, a list of the most likely causes of the patient's symptoms and physical findings. Based on the differential diagnosis, she orders the appropriate diagnostic tests, including blood and body fluid testing and X-rays. In some cases, she refers the patient to a specialist for diagnostic intervention.

Hurdles Between You and Diagnosis

As a patient, you can expect numerous hurdles in your pursuit of a definitive diagnosis. Over the next several pages, you'll find out what these are and how you can overcome them.

Doctors Cannot Feel Your Symptoms

Your doctor knows the science of medicine, but you know what feels normal or abnormal in your body. While describing your symptoms, keep in mind that symptoms are subjective and highly variable from one person to another. A broken hangnail on one person may feel like a broken arm to another. Your doctor does not know your pain threshold or your point of reference. You must describe your symptoms as specifically as possible.

When describing pain, use words such as sharp, dull, intermittent, *throbbing, stabbing,* or *searing.* Use metaphors, if necessary. If you have severe headaches, you might tell your doctor you feel as if your head is in a steel vise. If you have severe abdominal cramping, tell your doctor it feels as if Roto-Rooter is inside your intestines. Your goal is to help your doctor empathize and feel your symptoms. Give quantifiable examples whenever possible, and make sure your doctor understands how the symptoms affect your quality of life.

You Have a Large Stack of Records from Other Physicians Who Were Unable to Make a Diagnosis

The larger your stack of records, the more vulnerable you could be for a mental health label. In rare instances, a somatoform condition such as hypochondriasis or a conversion disorder can cause physical symptoms such as pain, cognitive impairment, or even paralysis. The online Physician Survey reveals that most physicians see somatoform conditions, malingering, or a desire to feed a drug addiction in 25 percent or fewer of their elusive cases. But they are often quick to conclude that a lengthy undiagnosed condition has a psychiatric cause and to suggest a full psychiatric workup. The psychiatric workup often suggests depression, a secondary condition that coexists with an undiagnosed chronic illness.

During one of my many mental-health evaluations during my quest for the correct medical diagnosis, I was labeled depressed. Of course I was depressed! Who wouldn't have been depressed given my circumstances? Depression was the result of my condition, not the cause. Although you cannot control your doctor's opinion, you can take steps to minimize the chances of an incorrect mental-health diagnosis. Your best defense is to appear calm and not highly emotional. The last thing you want to do is support your doctor's position that you suffer from a mental-health problem by having a meltdown during an office or hospital visit. You might find it helpful to present emotionally charged items in writing. You can also help your cause by taking charge of the situation right up front.

Present your case as a challenge to the doctor with a comment such as, "I realize none of the other doctors have been able to figure this out, but I've heard good things about you, and I'm hoping that you'll be the one to finally resolve this very complex case." A little flattery never hurts!

Doctors Have Biases Just Like Everyone Else

Five years ago, I encountered an emergency department physician who developed a healthy disdain for me before he even came into the exam room. Because I keep lists of medication, past hospitalizations and surgeries, and chronic conditions up to date on my computer, I printed them just before heading to the ER with severe abdominal pain. When this doctor viewed my file, he saw meticulous medical records, a copy of my Medicare card, and my age, which is lower than 65. He correctly concluded that I was receiving Social Security disability benefits and decided, based on my record-keeping ability and his own biases that, by golly, I was capable of working. He spent the better part of that hideous ER visit haranguing me and telling me, "You need to find a job," while I was doubled over in severe pain.

Although this example is extreme, physician biases do exist, simply because physicians are human. Your doctor may not seem to like you for reasons that have nothing to do with you as a person. He may feel inadequate if he is unable to find the right diagnosis and treatment, and he may direct this frustration toward you. Additionally, your proactive position might earn you the label of "difficult patient," so your behavior toward your doctor must be tempered with the utmost respect and appreciation. If you sense disrespect from your doctor in spite of your own respectful behavior, you probably need to find a different doctor. Regardless of whether or not you and your doctor like each other, you must have mutual respect in order to work together toward the common goals of diagnosis and treatment.

Your Doctor Has Probably Seen Other Patients in Worse Shape Than You

What seems like a major calamity to you may be business as usual for her. Although you are feeling miserable, totally debilitated, and at your wits' end, your doctor might think that you are lucky you don't have anything "serious." Doctors tend to consider life-threatening emergencies serious, and when they see them on a regular basis, they become desensitized to life-limiting conditions. Regardless of doctors' viewpoints, most would not have the audacity to make a trivializing comment directly to a patient.

However, one of the many specialists I consulted felt that he had a duty to tell me he had just completed rounds at the hospital and had seen patients my age (35 at the time) in much worse shape than I and went on to tell me that I was lucky I didn't have anything serious. As I sat there with my cane at my side, I told him I was sorry to hear that his other patients were suffering, but I did not pay my driver 12 dollars per hour to bring me to his office so that I could hear about their difficulties.

This level of offensive behavior is rare in the medical profession, and I hope you never have to endure it. But your doctor might rank your symptoms mentally against those of other patients on the "seriousness" scale and wonder why you are so upset when you don't have anything life-threatening. The best way to handle this is to present your case as calmly and factually as possible. Doctors are interested in facts, not drama. When you describe the effects of your symptoms on your quality of life, try to do so objectively and without self-pity, almost as if you are discussing your own patient. Your goal is to be taken as seriously as possible.

You and Your Doctor Are Not Speaking the Same Language

You may not be familiar with the many medical terms and acronyms your doctor uses. He is speaking "medical," and you are speaking English (Harding and Korsch 1998, 25).

Learning a New Language

If you are interested in increasing your knowledge of medicalese, you can read *The Patient's Guide to Medical Terminology* by Charlotte Isler or study *Medical Terminology: The Basics: Laminate Reference Chart* by Corinne B. Linton. The Medical Library Association has an excellent Web site called Deciphering Medspeak at www.mlanet.org/resources/medspeak, and you can also search www.medterms.com.

You must ask your doctor to explain anything that is not clear. Doctors are trained to be very scientific in their thinking, and this training directly affects their communication with patients.

Their scientific training also affects how they translate the medical history they receive from you into clinical terms. Following your office or hospital visit, your physician reads the notes from your conversation and tape records this information for entry into a report by a medical transcriptionist or by voice recognition software. The final report is put into your medical file and, in some cases, sent to other physicians. With each step that gets your medical history into the report, the margin for error increases. You must communicate all information to your doctor clearly and concisely in order to minimize the chance for errors during the first step in this process.

Medicine Is, at Its Core, an Uncertain Science

Every doctor makes mistakes in diagnosis and treatment (Groopman 2007, 7). An accurate diagnosis requires the expertise of doctors, nurses, X-ray technicians, and laboratory personnel, all of whom are fallible. Even when the nurses and lab or X-ray technicians do their jobs properly, they are dependent on the doctors' orders to know what to look for in their testing. If nurses or technicians don't do their jobs properly, you are vulnerable to errors such as lost samples or patient mix-ups. The doctor seeking the diagnostic testing depends on a radiologist to read X-ray films correctly.

With all the interdisciplinary cooperation required, the overall potential for error is scary. Among 1,087 individuals who received a battery of tests for prostate, ovarian, colorectal, and lung cancer in a cancer-screening trial, 43 percent had at least one false positive test result, according to Jennifer Elston Lafata, PhD, director of the Center for Health Services Research at the Henry Ford Hospital and the lead author on the study (Lafata 2004). If you have any inkling that a test result might not be accurate, don't be afraid to request a repeat of the test. Your doctor should repeat any test that shows a positive result for a life-threatening condition, and you should also get a second opinion. Finally, you can lower your risk of diagnostic errors by choosing a physician's office or hospital that uses electronic medical records.

Pathology, Lab, and X-Ray Reports Are Open to Interpretation

This fact created the emotional roller coaster that Laurie Todd endured during her deadly battle with cancer. The uncertainty of a pathology report creates additional emotional trauma to an already agonizing situation.

One doctor or radiologist can read an X-ray or pathology report as normal while another may interpret it as abnormal. Laboratory reports are even more convoluted because the normal range for a particular test can vary from one lab to another. Ideally, your doctor will weigh any questionable lab reports or X-rays, along with your history and symptoms, to determine what is normal or not normal for you.

Many Conditions Are Difficult to Diagnose Because of Limited Testing and Overlapping Symptoms

If you suffer from joint pain, brain fog, and fatigue, the cause of your symptoms could be any of a number of conditions, including fibromyalgia, Lyme disease, or lupus, to name just a few. To complicate things further, some of these conditions, such as fibromyalgia and chronic fatigue syndrome, coexist. Both fibromyalgia and chronic fatigue syndrome, along with Lyme disease, have limited testing, and some medical insurance plans do not cover the more sophisticated tests.

Another condition that deserves mention in this section is epilepsy. It is difficult to diagnose because many sufferers do not have seizures during testing and because there are other causes of seizures. Recent studies show that cardiovascular syncope (collapse resulting from disturbed heart rhythm) rather than epilepsy is the cause of 20 to 30 percent of seizures (Zaidi 2000, 181). One of the most serious commonly misdiagnosed conditions is ovarian cancer. The symptoms are very vague, and early diagnostic tools are less precise than more invasive procedures such as biopsies. (For a list of the one hundred most commonly misdiagnosed conditions, check out www.wrongdiagnosis.com/top-100.)

Your Doctor Doesn't Know What Is Wrong

If your doctor honestly has no idea what is causing your symptoms, the kindest and safest thing he can do is tell you, "I don't know." You are much better off hearing that than receiving an incorrect diagnosis or a blame-the-patient conclusion, such as, "It's all in your head" or, "It's stress-related." To a desperate patient, the wrong diagnosis seems better than none, but treatment for the wrong condition is risky at best. Your doctor may need to pull back the reins for your own safety when you are grasping at straws.

During my desperate search, I wanted to pursue anything and everything that might lead to a diagnosis and recovery. Fortunately, Dr. Wyatt was the voice of reason in the middle of all this turmoil. When I decided that my symptoms partially matched those of Chiari malformation, I wanted a referral to a neurosurgeon who specialized in this condition. Dr. Wyatt said, "No, that is too dangerous, and your symptoms don't match well enough to take that risk." Although he was honest and humble enough to say, "I don't know," he continued to help me seek answers and, at the same time, kept me from trying anything dangerous out of desperation.

Managed Care

Doctors are under tremendous pressure to keep costs down while increasing their patient load. With office visits averaging ten minutes or less, doctors and patients do not have adequate time together. You must present your case as quickly and concisely as possible. You must also do some research to determine which diagnostic tests you might need and be assertive in asking for them. The more vocal you are, the less likely your doctor is to surrender to cost-containment pressure from the health-care network. You may face even more resistance if you ask for a referral to an out-of-network specialist, but the extra battle is worth it if it leads to a correct diagnosis and treatment.

The Quest

The search for a diagnosis and treatment is akin to the search for that perfect job. It requires networking, research, preparation for office visits, and an image that will earn you the respect you need from the medical profession during this crucial time. You may find it unfair that you have to work so hard when you are already suffering physically, but anything in life that is worth having takes effort.

Your voice is one of your biggest assets in your quest for an accurate diagnosis and treatment. The more you share your story, the more clues you will gather from the people around you. The more you network, the more likely you are to hear, "I saw a lady on *Mystery Diagnosis, Dateline, Oprah*, and so on, whose symptoms are a lot like yours. She was diagnosed with…" I received many such clues throughout my journey, and I investigated each one thoroughly. You should leave no stone unturned during your quest for an accurate diagnosis and treatment. Your life, or at least your quality of life, depends on it.

The Internet is a gold mine for networking. You will find valuable clues while visiting message boards, forums, newsgroups, and support groups for conditions with symptoms similar to yours. Through the Internet, you have access to an infinite number of people who may have valuable information. You also have unlimited access to unsavory characters, so be careful. As with any online activity, use caution when sharing information about yourself. It is one thing to share symptoms, but be careful with personal information such as addresses, phone numbers, marital status, and number of children in your household.

Whether you network by word of mouth or online, you must make every effort to get your story out there. The more you share your story, the more likely you are to stumble upon the correct diagnosis and treatment. Remember, a chance conversation with a neighbor set in motion the chain of events that led to my recovery. You must not discount any possible clue, no matter how dubious it may seem.

Networking and research have complementary roles in the search for a diagnosis. The information you gather from networking may give you direction for your research. When someone tells you, "I read about a case just like yours," God has opened a door for you and given you a new direction for your research.

You will find the research portion of your search absolutely daunting. You have the Internet, bookstores, and libraries at your disposal. Where do you begin? Once again, the Internet is a wealth of information. Keep in mind, though, that not all Web sites are built or maintained by reputable individuals or organizations. A legitimate Web site will include up-to-date information and the qualifications of the author. It should identify the source of its information, along with facts and figures and links to other sites for additional information. It should not contain advertisements or suggest one specific treatment plan. URLs ending in *.com* are typically associated with commercial sites; those ending in *.net* are typically Internet networks; those ending in *.gov* are government organizations; those ending in *.edu* are affiliated with educational institutions; and those ending in *.org* are usually nonprofit organizations. Your best bets for reliable information are the *.edu* and *.gov* sites (Oz 2006, 242-43).

Helpful Resources for Diagnosis

To search for conditions that match your symptoms, visit medlineplus.gov or webapps.jhu.edu/jhuniverse/medicine/diseases, and click on conditions you think may be causing your symptoms. If you suspect a rare illness, you can search www.rarediseases.org. If you would like to search by symptoms to see which medical conditions match, you can visit www.wrongdiagnosis .com or symptomchecker.aarp.org. To learn more about diagnostic tests you may need, visit www.health.harvard.edu/diagnostic-tests.

Helpful hard-copy reference guides include *The Merck Manual of Diagnosis and Therapy* by Robert S. Porter, Thomas V. Jones, and Mark H. Beer and *Symptom to Diagnosis* by Scott D.C. Stern, Diane Altkorn, and Adam Cifu. Books on specific conditions are available online and through libraries and bookstores. For cost savings, check out eBay, Amazon.com's and ABE.com's used books, and used book stores. If you live near a medical school, try the medical library. Medical librarians have valuable experience directing both medical personnel and lay persons in the right direction for information. Medical libraries are also a great place to network. For online medical research, visit the National Library of Medicine at www.nlm.nih.gov.

You can use your Web browser to search, using keywords that include suspected or related medical conditions or your symptoms. You may find that each search leads to another, then another, and next thing you know, several hours have gone by. Although you may not have found an answer, you will have ruled out a number of possibilities, so you're still ahead of the game. And the more searches you do, the better your chances are of stumbling onto that golden nugget of information that will give you back your life.

You should present your Internet research and your medical history to your doctor during your office visit. Use caution when presenting your research because the medical community has little patience for "armchair doctors." Don't treat the information from the Internet as if it trumps your doctor's years of training and experience. Your input can be helpful, and your doctor may appreciate your help as long as you present it properly and respect her position as the medical expert.

Your overall presentation has a significant effect on how seriously you are taken. Your doctor is looking at other things besides history. She is observing your demeanor and mannerisms for possible clues. Your goal is to be as calm, articulate, and respectful as possible. Make it clear that you are actively participating in your diagnosis and recovery but at the same time, you need and appreciate your doctor's help. As Dr. Phil would say, you must "inspire" your doctor to want to help you.

All of this effort may seem overwhelming...and yes, it can be a full-time job. But if you are suffering from an undiagnosed condition, with a 5 percent chance of a full recovery, the pursuit of a correct diagnosis may be the most important job of your life.

My Mom's Battle

In early 2006, my mom began to experience sporadic medical issues, beginning with heart palpitations so severe that she had to be hospitalized and referred to a cardiologist for testing. While undergoing testing for the chest pain, physicians discovered that Mom had a hiatal hernia, and later, an inguinal hernia. She underwent surgery to correct the inguinal hernia and began taking medication for the hiatal hernia discomfort.

By late 2006, this beautiful, sweet lady was suffering with more pronounced nausea, abdominal pain, difficulty swallowing solid food, and weight loss. A blood test revealed anemia, which most likely had caused her heart palpitations earlier. Mom's diagnosis was delayed because her symptoms were treated as individual medical issues when, in fact, they were important clues to one very devastating underlying cause.

By the time Mom was referred to a surgical specialist for more thorough testing three months later, she had trouble swallowing most foods and even some liquids. The surgical specialist immediately scheduled an esophagram, a series of X-rays of the esophagus, for the next morning. The esophagram revealed a severe esophageal stricture, the cause of Mom's difficulty in swallowing. The next day, her esophagus closed completely, and she was hospitalized for three-and-a-half weeks.

During Mom's hospitalization, we received the devastating news that she had esophageal cancer and that her esophagus was completely closed and undilatable. A subsequent test showed that the cancer had metastasized to her liver. The surgical oncologist gave Mom a prognosis of 8 to 12 months. He stated that if she had had an endoscopy (an internal scope of the gastrointestinal tract) several months earlier, her chances would have been better.

Mom immediately launched a valiant battle against stage IV esophageal cancer. She welcomed chemotherapy treatments along with alternative treatments. Despite the agony of five months with a closed esophagus, Mom's spirits remained high, her positive attitude unwavering. She did not let the closed esophagus inhibit her enjoyment of food; she chewed everything she could get her hands on and then discreetly disposed of it. She sat outside on the swing Dad bought for her and enjoyed the nice weather. She saw her downtime as an opportunity to do a lot of reading, and she delighted in the 280 get-well cards she received. She even made a list of all the things that made her happy. Mom was determined to enjoy whatever time she had left, and she maintained her beautiful smile throughout her courageous fight. Cancer had found a formidable foe.

After five months, her large tumor had softened enough to allow the insertion of a stent into her esophagus. The stent allowed her to take in liquids and soft foods. For the most part this improved her quality of life, and she forged on with chemotherapy for another four months. During this time, she made numerous trips to the emergency room for fever and difficulty with her feeding tube.

Then her oncologist delivered the bad news that the cancer was spreading. He recommended cessation of chemotherapy and an emphasis on palliative care to keep Mom as comfortable as possible. She took this news like a champ and immediately added more alternative treatments to her regimen, still determined to beat the cancer. She never talked about dying or the end of her life. She always took the position that she was going to beat the cancer. She remained upbeat for Dad, my brothers, and me, and she tried to minimize our sadness and concern.

By February 2008, we could see that Mom was beginning to slip away. The hospitalizations were more frequent, and she was getting weaker. She surpassed the doctors' prognosis of eight to twelve months when she reached the one-year mark on March 12, 2008, but we knew she didn't have much time left. On April 15, Mom came home from the hospital for the last time. When the emergency medical service personnel transported her from the ambulance into the house, she looked up at her beloved home and smiled. It was at the top of her happy list. Within hours, she slipped into a coma. On April 16, a hospice nurse predicted that Mom would not live past 9:00 p.m. Mom, always one to have the final say in her quiet dignified manner, took her last breath at 9:15 p.m. She was just 67 years old.

As you can see, an accurate and timely diagnosis is critical. It can mean the difference between life and death or, at the very least, quality of life versus misery. As someone who has seen the life-threatening and life-limiting consequences of misdiagnosis, I implore you to stop at nothing to get the correct diagnosis and treatment.

Chapter 2

Head It Off at the Pass, Part One

Strengthening Your System

The best way to manage an illness or an injury is to prevent it in the first place or, at the very least, minimize the damage with early detection. Medication and surgery greatly improve the quality of our lives and may even save them, but they also carry a number of risks. What if we could avoid medication or surgery altogether with a healthy lifestyle?

Help from a Healthy Lifestyle

Steven Alexander went to a doctor recently for the first time in 40 years. Aside from an occasional cold or the flu, he had not had any medical problems. He was seeking medical help at last because he could no longer control his blood pressure with a healthy lifestyle, and it had risen to a dangerous level. While I'm not advocating staying out of doctors' offices for years at a time, I wanted to learn how he has remained healthy without any medical intervention for so long.

Steven describes himself as a self-taught naturopath and homeopath who looks to a healthy lifestyle for illness prevention and healing. He seeks natural medical guidance from Life Extension, a natural health organization with a large medical advisory board. He purchases nutritional supplements from them, and he also takes advantage of the organization's laboratory tests that help determine his unique nutritional needs. He advocates a diet based on biblical principles and insists that our bodies were not engineered to ingest processed food. He believes that our instincts are toward the outdoors and that we should live off the land. He even goes as far as to say that we are killing ourselves with processed food.

Steven regularly eats a diet rich in cancer-fighting plant sterols, whole grains, nuts, yogurt, eggs, fish, chicken, and turkey. He is a big fan of blueberries because of their antioxidant properties, along with walnuts and oatmeal for their effect on cholesterol. He also advocates regular exercise and a youthful, positive attitude to complete a healthy lifestyle.

Steven brings up a good point with his diet based on biblical principles. In the book of Daniel, chapter 1, Daniel and his men were ordered to eat the Babylonian king's royal food while in captivity to gain physical and intellectual strength in preparation for servitude. But Daniel requested a vegetable diet with only water to drink instead of the rich meats and wine ordered by the king. The king's men were afraid to disobey orders, so Daniel asked for a ten-day trial of the vegetable-and-water diet. At the end of the ten days, Daniel and his men were physically stronger and continued to grow in knowledge and wisdom.

Jordan Rubin concurs in his book *Patient, Heal Thyself.* Rubin suffered from Crohn's disease so severely that he nearly died. His weight plunged to 104 pounds, and at the worst point he overheard nurses crying in the hospital hallway, with one predicting that he would not live through the night. By this time, he had consulted numerous doctors, and his only medical options were radical surgery to remove all of his large and part of his small intestine or J-pouch surgery, an experimental procedure at that time. Instead, Rubin opted for a natural solution and consulted a nutritionist who believed healing was possible with a diet based upon biblical principles. Rubin moved temporarily to be near the nutritionist and learn how to adopt this healing diet. Within three months he had made dramatic improvement and gained over 50 pounds. His Crohn's disease went into remission, and he wrote 19 books based on his experiences and his nutritional research (Rubin 2002, 15-29).

As you can see, a healthy lifestyle is very powerful. Gastroenterologist Joseph Brasco, MD, coauthored five books with Rubin, and he offers a pyramid analogy when seeking healing and maintaining optimal health. First, we must exhaust all opportunities to heal with a healthy diet, adequate rest, a healthy outlet for stress, and regular exercise. If these options do not help the symptoms, the next step is to add a trial of vitamins or supplements. If still not successful, then try prescription medication, with the last resort being surgery. Dr. Brasco takes his pledge to first do no harm very seriously, opting for treatments with the fewest side effects or risks first.

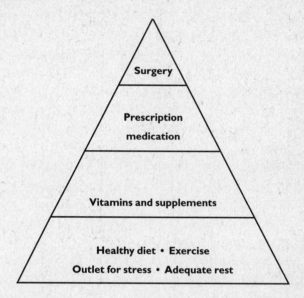

Eating Healthy

So what exactly is a healthy diet? Open 20 different magazines, and you will probably find 20 different articles with different opinions, although you may find some commonalities. I interviewed a number of physicians, alternative practitioners, and wellness professionals, and with some variations, they all agreed that a healthy diet should include whole foods, limited animal protein, whole grains, fruits and vegetables, healthy fats, lean protein, and plenty of water.

Several alternative practitioners recommended stricter guidelines that limit a healthy diet to pure water or herbal tea; 50 percent raw foods that include nine servings of fruits and vegetables per day; limited free-range, grass-fed, hormone-free meat; fish with low mercury counts; limited or no dairy; nuts and other healthy fats; limited or no whole grains; tofu;

no additives; no preservatives; and only honey and stevia for sweeteners. Say what? Oh, no! What about Starbucks?

Good news, Starbucks fans! A healthy diet does not have to be quite that restrictive. In fact, coffee offers protection against diabetes, gallstones, Parkinson's disease, and kidney disease. If you choose to go dairy-free, you can have your latte made with soy milk, or you can try rice or almond milk. Low fat and skim milk are good choices if you include dairy products in your diet. Additionally, a recent study suggests that caffeine may offer protection against skin cancer (Heffernan 2009). Chocolate lovers can also rejoice. Dark chocolate contains cancer-fighting antioxidants and cocoa phenols that lower blood pressure. But remember, moderation is the key. No binging, just nibbling. Ditto for coffee. Too much caffeine leads to dehydration.

A healthy diet should be doable and affordable. If you set the bar too high, you may get discouraged and find solace at the nearest fast-food restaurant. According to internist Celia Lloyd-Turney, MD, the biggest reasons for failing to maintain a healthy lifestyle are cost and time.

But a healthy lifestyle is attainable, say Ivy Larson and Andrew Larson, MD, authors of *The Gold Coast Cure*. Their all-inclusive lifestyle plan reduces the inflammation that causes conditions such as asthma, allergies, fibromyalgia, and multiple sclerosis. The program also reduces cholesterol, blood pressure, and triglycerides. The Larsons' mission is to make a healthy lifestyle possible for the average busy family with budget constraints. They accomplish this with healthy, time-saving recipes in their *Whole Foods Diet Cookbook* and with a 30-minute workout in their book *Firmer, Fitter, Faster*. Their Web site, www.the2larsons.com, features video clips packed with helpful tips on nutritious food choices and efficient exercise routines.

The Challenges

Healthy foods do not have to be expensive. Beans, nuts, tofu, tempeh, ground flaxseeds, whole grains, and canned salmon are excellent examples of inexpensive whole foods (food that is processed as little as possible). Frozen fruits and vegetables are also great sources of nutrition. While selecting a bag of frozen blueberries during a recent trip to the grocery store, I was pleased to see just one ingredient listed on the bag—blueberries. No preservatives or sugar, just blueberries.

The grocery store is not the only source of inexpensive healthy food. A wonderful program called Angel Food Ministries makes healthy food available at affordable prices. They sell a box of food that would normally cost $60 for $30. This nondenominational program is open to anyone regardless of income and operates out of churches in communities across the country. (For more information, visit www.angelfoodministries.com.) Many communities have food banks for people who cannot afford to purchase food or who do not have Angel Food Ministries available.

Senior citizens have a particularly difficult time maintaining a healthy diet. Their fixed incomes do not always allow for both healthy food and necessary medications, particularly when they fall prey to the infamous Medicare Part D "donut hole." Seniors with debilitating medical conditions are often unable to prepare healthy meals even if they have the food. In addition to Angel Food Ministries, which offers a Senior/Convenience package, seniors can take advantage of inexpensive meals at senior centers or the Meals on Wheels program.

Children also face unique nutritional challenges because they are at the mercy of factors over which they have no control. They may have limited access to healthy foods because of their family's financial situation or because of poor nutritional habits caused by a frenzied family lifestyle or lack of knowledge about healthy eating. Childhood obesity has skyrocketed in the U.S. because of the availability of convenience foods and busy but sedentary lifestyles. Sadly, obese children become obese, unhealthy adults.

Fortunately, balanced lunches are available in most public schools free or at a reduced cost for those who cannot pay full price. In some communities, children who qualify can receive free, balanced lunches during the summer at recreation centers. Families who have the financial means to buy healthy food but not the time to prepare it may benefit from one of the many meal assembly services popping up across the country. These services allow clients to prepare healthy meals based on recipes selected by the service, using ingredients prepared by the service (for example, chopped vegetables), and utensils cleaned by the service.

If you are committed to preparing healthy meals, at the end of this chapter you will find some basic guidelines to keep in mind while shopping for and preparing food. Though a healthy diet can seem like a lot of work, the results are well worth it. According to Kevin Ready, the Huntsville Hospital Wellness Center's program manager, type 2 diabetes is 90 percent preventable and, with the right lifestyle changes that include a healthy diet and exercise regimen, highly manageable. Alternative and allopathic practitioners agree with Kevin's assessment. Recent studies yield the same feedback (Hu 2001). A healthy diet can prevent other diseases such as cancer, heart disease, osteoporosis, and arthritis.

Weighing Down Your Joints

Obesity prevention and reversal are key factors in the treatment of a number of diseases, particularly arthritis. In fact, when I sought a veterinary specialist's help for my German shepherd's hip dysplasia, he told me that weight was the number-one factor in joint afflictions. He then looked at me and said, "It works that way for humans too."

I guess he could see that Beau was not getting to McDonald's, Burger King, Arby's, and Hardee's by himself. Beau has since slimmed down, thanks to a weight-management prescription food. And we have both backed off the fast food. Beau is now a svelte 80 pounds, and his hip dysplasia symptoms are noticeably better. Before his weight loss, his age in human years was 64; now it is 55, evidence that weight loss can help us regain some of our youth.

Specific Dietary Needs

If you have a condition such as high blood pressure, high cholesterol, diabetes, arthritis, or osteoporosis or if you have a high risk for cancer, I recommend that you ask your physician for a referral to a nutritionist to help you design a diet to fit your specific needs for prevention or reversal. Nutritionists know which foods have too much unhealthy fat, salt, and cholesterol, and they also know which nutrients you need for your particular situation. Ideally, you will receive most of your vital nutrients from healthy foods.

Supplements are just what the term suggests—they supplement your diet. They are an adjunct therapy designed to complement a healthy diet. But even a healthy diet needs support, because some nutrient levels are nearly impossible to achieve with diet alone, particularly the omega-3 family. Dr. Brasco recommends a daily regimen of vitamin E and fish oil supplementation for a better ratio of omega-3 fatty acids to the less healthy omega-6 fatty acids. He also recommends a daily probiotic supplement for everyone. In his book, *The Probiotic Diet*, Dr. Brasco describes how the vast majority of autoimmune disorders originate in the gastrointestinal tract. When there are not enough healthy bacteria present, the GI tract becomes a gateway to inflammation. Daily probiotic supplementation helps feed healthy bacteria to the GI tract.

Of course, a healthy diet is also key to a happy gut. As a holistic practitioner, Martha Whitney has seen the path of destruction left in the gut by unhealthy foods. Too many overprocessed, highly refined foods cause the mucus build-up that is a hotbed for so many illnesses. The good news is, Martha has seen a great deal of improvement in those who are willing to adopt a healthier diet.

If you are getting annual physicals, then your doctor will check some of your vitamin levels, such as B-12, as part of your evaluation. Your standard evaluation may not include testing for vitamin D levels, even though recent studies show that many of us are deficient. In fact, Dr. Phillip Watkins has found that 80 percent of his mitral valve prolapse and autonomic disorders patients are vitamin D–deficient. Vitamin D deficiency has been linked to conditions such as osteoporosis, depression, diabetes, cancer, heart disease (Holick 2007), and more recently, multiple sclerosis (Goodin 2009). If you are interested in vitamin D testing, you may need to request a specialized test from your physician.

If your diet is not rich in antioxidants, you may want to consider a supplement. According to the National Cancer Institute, antioxidants may slow or prevent the development of cancer. Additionally, a recent study found that the antioxidants in one glass of wine per day may lower the risk of Barrett's esophagus, a precursor to esophageal cancer (Preidt 2009).

Reviews are mixed on antioxidants as a preventive for heart disease, but the American Heart Association recommends getting antioxidants from food, rather than from supplements. It cites red wine and grape juice as sources of flavonoids, a type of antioxidant.

Exercise Is Essential

A healthy diet is only part of the equation. Exercise is essential for preventing and reversing obesity and related diseases, and as a nation, we need this. The Centers for Disease Control estimate that 46.2 percent of the population is insufficiently active and that obesity-related illnesses cost an estimated $98 billion to $129 billion. About 80 percent of obese adults suffer from diabetes, high cholesterol levels, and coronary artery disease.

According to Brian Hall, Certified Personal Trainer, the benefits of a balanced exercise program are invaluable and include...

- increased energy levels that help in job performance and in every area of life
- stress management and relief from depression
- stronger immune system, resulting in better overall health
- reduced chance of type 2 diabetes because of stable blood sugar and increased cellular sensitivity to insulin
- heart disease prevention with raising of good cholesterol, lowering of blood pressure, and prevention of dangerous plaque by opening up blood vessels
- cancer prevention, with consistent exercise slashing the risk of colorectal, breast, and ovarian cancers by 30 to 50 percent
- osteoporosis prevention, with weight-bearing exercise, such as running, hiking, weight lifting, some types of yoga and Pilates, and stair climbing that build bone density (any activity that forces your muscles to work against gravity is helpful)
- increased longevity, with consistent physical activity cutting the risk of premature death by 50 percent

Hall also cites several medical conditions that a balanced exercise program improves:

- *Muscular dystrophy.* Research shows that strength training decreases the level of muscle weakness associated with this disease.

- *Arthritis.* Regular exercise builds the muscles around the joints, and this in turn lubricates the joints.

- *Osteoporosis.* Weight-bearing or resistance training strengthens the muscles around the weakened bones, leading to better bone density.

- *Obesity.* A good balance of weight resistance training combined with cardiovascular training is especially important in treating obesity. This balance provides optimal fat-burning capabilities.

- *Type 2 diabetes.* This condition is reversible with a healthy diet and an exercise program that improves blood glucose control and overall metabolism.

- *Cardiovascular disease.* Cardiac rehab patients benefit from a combination strength-training and cardiovascular-training regimen.

- *Cancer.* Walking programs have been shown to help patients with localized cancer by slowing the disease's progression. With some cancers, strength training is beneficial.

As you can see, a balanced exercise program is critical in meeting nearly everyone's fitness needs. Unless you have a medical condition that dictates otherwise, you need a regular exercise program that combines cardiovascular training with strength training. If you prefer to work out in a gym, an efficient program starts with a five- to ten-minute cardio warm-up on a bike, Stairmaster, or treadmill, then a set of repetitions (12 to 15) for each major muscle group on weight equipment, such as Nautilus, and then more cardio (20 to 30 minutes) after the strength training.

If you move quickly from one exercise to the next, you can keep your heart rate up for maximum cardio and fat-burning benefits. Speaking of fat-burning, strength training is just as important as cardio for revving up your metabolism. You need both.

Inexpensive Options for Physical Fitness

What if you can't afford a gym? Check online or in the government pages of the phone book for a municipal parks and recreation program. These programs vary from one community to another, depending on resources. Some facilities are free and have basic equipment; others charge a small fee and are like health clubs, with trainers available. I am fortunate to live in a city with a great parks and recreation program. I work out in a nice facility less than two miles from my home. It has a full line of Nautilus equipment, free weights, treadmills, and exercise bikes—and it's all free.

If you don't like weight equipment, you can still get a great cardio and strength-training workout with certain kinds of yoga or with a Pilates mat or reformer workout.* These workouts get the heart rate up with movements that flow quickly from one to the next. They also provide great resistance training since you support your body weight in many of the poses.

For more information on physical fitness, visit www.acsm.org and click on General Public in the Resources For column. You will find a wealth of information, including guidelines suggesting that you engage in moderate-level exercise for at least 30 minutes at least five times per week. These guidelines are in line with those of the American Cancer Society and the American Heart Association. Even if your schedule does not permit five workouts a week, you can still benefit from three per week, according to personal trainers Brian Hall and Ivy Larson. The secret is to make your workouts as efficient as possible with compounded movements, or movements that work

---

* If you prefer a Christian alternative to yoga, check out www.PraiseMoves.com.

multiple muscle groups. A certified fitness professional can show you how to do this safely.

Designed to Move

What kind of exercise should you choose? Simple answer—that which you are most likely to do *consistently*. Which time of day is best for exercise? The time when you are most likely to exercise. In other words, you must find an exercise program that you enjoy and that fits your lifestyle. Be sure to check with your physician before embarking on a new fitness journey, and make sure that your fitness instructor has the proper credentials. Look for a bachelor's degree in exercise science or physiology or a personal trainer certification. Seventy-plus organizations certify personal trainers, and many of these organizations are very good. Ask your fitness instructor about his training, his preparation for certification, and his years of experience as a trainer. If properly trained, your instructor will emphasize proper form when showing you how to use weight equipment or how to perform yoga or Pilates poses.

Our bodies were designed for exercise and for movement in general. When we don't listen to them and when we force them to do something counterintuitive, we risk injury. When we are sporadic with our activity, we get into trouble. Think about the weekend warrior syndrome. Our bodies are not intended to sit 40 hours per week and then engage in heavy exercise or yardwork during the weekend. In fact, our bodies were not designed to sit for 40 hours per week, period. Prolonged sitting is the number-one cause of spinal degeneration.

But combine continuous sitting with sporadic heavy physical activity, and we have bigger problems. How many times have you circled the parking lot at a shopping center, looking for the closest parking space on a beautiful sunny day instead of taking advantage of the opportunity for some light walking and vitamin D? As natural pharmacist Terry Wingo says, "The problem is that we drive to the gym, and we ride a lawnmower." His point is that we fail to take advantage of opportunities for moderate, ongoing activity that will give us a better foundation for heavy activity.

Moving the Right Way

Surgery and medication are often preventable if we move the way our bodies are designed to move, according to ergonomics expert Alan Hedge, PhD, and Anthony Houssain, DC. We need to understand how to use our bodies, something most of us do not think about until we are already injured. And once the pain starts, we want to treat the pain rather than the root cause.

But if we don't treat the root cause, we cannot expect the pain to stay away. Dr. Houssain recommends using stronger areas of the body to compensate for weaker ones and to shift weight, if needed. For example, lifting with the hips and not the back can help to avoid injury. He also suggests anticipating activities that may tax the body and preparing accordingly, such as a weekend spent gardening or moving furniture or even riding in a car for an extended period. You can take steps to ensure proper back support for these activities and also schedule frequent breaks.

Dr. Hedge sees a large number of repetitive-motion injuries and believes they are 100 percent preventable. The most common work-related injury is low back pain from lifting incorrectly or prolonged sitting. Disabling work-related injuries include back problems, carpal tunnel syndrome, reflex sympathetic dystrophy, and vibration white finger. Attention to ergonomics can prevent and improve many of these problems. Sometimes the solution is as simple as an adjustment in chair height.

Ergonomics is just as important in the home as in the workplace, especially for children. Because their bones are still forming, children run the risk of bone deformation from ergonomic injuries. The most common activities at home that cause ergonomic injuries include computer use, video-game use, gardening, home improvement, baking, cleaning, and shoveling snow. Any activity done to excess creates an opportunity for injury.

Dr. Hedge recommends lifting no more than 25 pounds, and he believes 50 pounds is cause for worry. Mothers should carry infants and small children on the hip or in a sling carrier and use strollers as much as possible. For comprehensive information on how you can protect you and your family from ergonomic injuries, you can visit Dr. Hedge's Web site at www.ergo.human.cornell.edu. This site has an abundance of information, with guidelines for workstations, computer use, computer keyboards, parents, and children, with a number of self-tests that ask you where it hurts.

If you treat your body well, it is more likely to serve you well. You must be conscious of what you put into it and of the demands you place on it. Think of your body as a car. Would you put low-grade gasoline into a brand-new Ferrari? Would you allow your Ferrari to sit idle for weeks or months at a time? Would you drive with the parking brake on or leave the lights on while it's parked? Your body deserves much greater respect than an automobile. You only have one body—treat it well.

Basic Guidelines for Selecting and Preparing Food

Aim for five to nine servings per day of fruits and vegetables. This is easier than it sounds. You can consume several servings in a healthy salad or in a marinara sauce with vegetables.

Eat a rainbow of colors. No, this does not mean M&Ms or Skittles! Try to select whole foods in as many different colors as possible. Think strawberries, blueberries, oranges, melons, different-colored bell peppers, broccoli, carrots, sweet potatoes, and squash.

Buy organic, if possible. If your budget will not accommodate organic foods, the next best thing for produce is a fruit-and-vegetable wash to remove pesticides.

Select food with the fewest ingredients and ingredients with the fewest syllables. You will find most of these products in the outer perimeter of your grocery store. Try to avoid ingredients ending in "ose."

Eat meat sparingly. It takes three or four days to break down in the body, stressing the liver and other organs. Meat—particularly red meat and processed meat—has been linked to increased risk for several cancers, especially colon cancer.

Select the healthiest protein sources possible. Animal proteins carry a number of risks. Farmers treat conventionally raised farm animals living in cramped quarters with antibiotics to reduce the risk of infection. When these antibiotics are passed on to us in our food supply, we risk becoming antibiotic resistant. Free-range farm animals are allowed to roam and do not need antibiotics. Grass-fed animals are also healthier because they have not been fed animal by-products. Hormone-free farm animals are much safer for us to eat since they haven't been given the hormones that can increase our cancer risk. Look for terms such as "grass-fed," "free-range," "certified antibiotic," and "USDA certified organic" when selecting meat products. Meat-free protein sources abound in the form of tofu, tempeh, and beans.

Select fish with low levels of mercury and high levels of omega-3 fatty acids. Omega-3 fatty acids have a number of health benefits, but high mercury levels can cause symptoms such as lethargy, inability to concentrate, irritability, and numbness and tingling in the extremities. For a listing of both in a variety of seafood choices, visit www.americanheart.org/presenter.jhtml?identifier=3013797.

Select the healthiest dairy products. Dairy has long been considered a source of calcium, which has been shown in some studies to reduce the risk of osteoporosis. But most of the alternative practitioners I consulted and some of the allopathic practitioners believe that the risks associated with dairy outweigh the benefits. The concerns they cited include antibiotic and estrogen levels in dairy products, fat content in some dairy sources, adverse effects on the immune system, and changing properties as a result of pasteurization and homogenization.

But there are ways to enjoy dairy while modifying the risks. Fermented dairy sources such as yogurt and kefir are healthier options. Hormone-free dairy products remove the estrogen issue and low-fat products reduce the unhealthy fats associated with many dairy products.

If you do not have a dairy-rich diet, there are other steps you can take toward osteoporosis prevention. Tobacco products and soft drinks erode bone tissue. Eliminating these products can help reduce osteoporosis, along with weight-bearing exercise, adequate vitamin D intake and calcium-rich plant sources, particularly leafy green vegetables.

Know your fats. Not all fats are bad. The worst is trans fat, found in fried food, cookies, crackers, chips, and shortening. Saturated fat, found in red meat and vegetable oil, is also unhealthy but not quite to the extent of trans fat. A much better choice is polyunsaturated fat, found in flaxseed oil, fish, and walnuts. Monounsaturated fatty acids are the healthiest, and you can find them in olive oil, canola oil, almonds, avocados, and dark chocolate.

Eliminate white flour in favor of whole wheat flour or white wheat flour. Replace unhealthy starches with whole grains such as oatmeal, brown rice, quinoa, and whole wheat pasta. These foods add fiber for fullness and reduce the risk of heart disease and diabetes.

Plan ahead. Prepare a list before you go to the grocery store, determine what you will eat before you become ravenous, and review nutritional information for restaurants online before you go to them. Advance planning can make the difference between a healthy meal and a binge.

Watch sugar and sweetener intake. Try to limit products containing corn syrup. Replace granulated sugar with lower-calorie, less-processed turbinado sugar. Consider the dangers of artificial sweeteners: Aspartame has been linked to a number of neurological disorders; saccharin testing has revealed bladder cancer in laboratory rats; and sucralose, the newest artificial sweetener, may cause side effects such as skin rashes, dizziness, and intestinal cramping. Stevia and agave nectar, both natural substances, are safer alternatives. The major soft drink companies are developing diet drinks sweetened with stevia; although the stevia is less toxic, the drinks will still contain additives and coloring though.

Stay hydrated. Water makes up 65 to 75 percent of the body and is necessary for your systems to function properly. To maintain a proper level of hydration and flush away toxins, you must drink six to

eight glasses of water per day. Plain water is the most efficient way to
replace lost body fluids, followed by unsweetened fruit or vegetable
juices diluted with water or seltzer water. With a plethora of water
choices available, which should you choose—mineral, distilled, spar-
kling, or artesian? According to Linda Rector-Page, author of *Healthy
Healing*, all of these choices are all healthier than tap water, although
she recommends distilled water for healing (Rector-Page 1992, 63).
However, several of the physicians I interviewed maintain that municipal tap water is safe and that the amount of toxicity is negligible, far
less than in soft drinks.

Chapter 3

Head It Off at the Pass, Part Two

Reducing Your Risk Factors

As you've seen in chapter 2, any positive lifestyle change takes discipline and effort. Addictions, however, present unique challenges, and among the most difficult are alcohol, illicit drugs, and smoking. All of these carry significant risks, and you should address them even before diet and exercise.

Where to Start

Changing one unhealthy behavior is difficult enough; changing more than one at a time is setting the bar a little high and can result in discouragement. Start with the most perilous first. Addictions to drugs, alcohol, and smoking present risks not only to those with the addictions, but to others as well. Drug and alcohol addictions create a number of dangers to others, particularly the traffic hazards imposed by impaired drivers. Scientists believe that secondhand smoke creates a health risk for others. The Centers for Disease Control conducted a three-year study after a smoking ban in Pueblo, Colorado, and found that hospitalizations for heart attack dropped 41 percent, suggesting that secondhand smoke may cause heart disease. (To view the CDC report on this study, visit www.cdc.gov/mmwr/preview/mmwrhtml/mm5751a1.htm.)

As the American Heart Association points out, smoking is a risk factor for heart disease that can be changed. The AHA measures the risk of coronary heart disease for smokers as two to four times more than for nonsmokers. But heart disease is not the only risk. While interviewing numerous physicians and nurses, I asked all of them which risk factor is most causative for cancer. Without hesitation, they all said, "Smoking." Tobacco use is a risk factor for cancers of the lung, mouth, esophagus, bladder, cervix, pancreas, and other areas of the body. In fact, the American Cancer Society devotes a large section of its Web site to smoking cessation support. The good news is that the risk drops after tobacco use has ceased.

If you are interested in smoking cessation, you have a number of resources from which to choose. However, your most powerful tool is your own will. You have to want to stop smoking, and until you make that commitment, that conscious decision to stop, all the patches and nicotine gum in the world will not help. Think about your loved ones who need you. The Centers for Disease Control and Prevention estimate that smoking shortens adult males' lifespan by an average of 13.2 years and that of adult females by an average of 14.5 years.

Care of Teeth and Gums

Smoking and heavy drinking (and also dehydration) cause plaque and tartar build-up that leads to or worsens periodontal (gum) disease. Recent studies have shown a correlation between periodontal disease and heart disease. Periodontal disease is an inflammatory disease that is associated with other inflammatory conditions such as diabetes, rheumatoid arthritis, and kidney disease.

To learn more and to take the risk assessment test for periodontal disease, visit the American Academy of Periodontology at www.perio.org and click on the Gum Disease tab. Warning signs of periodontal disease include swollen, bleeding gums and pain or tenderness, although this disease can be asymptomatic. If you are taking medication that causes dryness in the mouth, the decreased saliva flow can increase your chances of getting periodontal disease or tooth decay. If you already have diabetes, you are vulnerable to a much faster progression of gum disease.

Aside from disease prevention, there are other reasons for maintaining good oral hygiene, including regular cleanings by your dentist every six months. Tartar results from plaque, and tartar causes bad breath. Nobody wants that. More important, your dentist is your first line of defense against oral cancer. Because she is the one who examines your mouth, she will probably catch any sign of oral cancer before your physician. And she just might save your life in the event of an abscess. In rare cases, an infected tooth can be fatal if the abscess goes to the brain.

Managing Medications

Medication management is a huge proactive step toward the prevention of illness, injury, or even premature death. Both inpatient and outpatient medication errors are preventable. Chapter 6 addresses hospital medication errors, along with other inpatient safety issues. Throughout the interview process for this book, I asked a number of medical practitioners and patient safety specialists which type of medical error (for example, surgery, medication, laboratory, X-ray) is most dangerous. They all said, "Medication errors."

The consequences range from inconvenience to death, with a number of outcomes in between. Six percent of all emergency department admissions are the result of adverse events caused by medication errors. The tragic death of actor Heath Ledger spotlights the worst-case scenario. Ledger died from an accidental overdose of six different prescription medications that never should have been combined. Somewhere along the way, this dangerous combination went undetected by a physician and a pharmacy.

When I asked Dr. Wyatt which medications are the most dangerous, he replied, "All of them are dangerous if prescribed or taken incorrectly." The opportunities for dangerous errors are vast when you consider all of the steps between the pharmaceutical company, physician, pharmacy, and patient. The first step includes development of the medication and its bulk manufacturing and transport to pharmacies. Pharmaceutical representatives visit physicians to market their companies' drugs. Remember, your

PCP is seeing 25 to 50 patients per day, so she depends on pharmaceutical reps for education on the latest medications.

When you visit your doctor, she writes a prescription for the medication she believes you need, based at least in part on inputs from the reps. You look at the prescription, cannot read it, and take it to your pharmacy, hoping that your pharmacist can read it. And what do those mysterious scribbles mean anyway? (If you would like to learn more about prescription shorthand, visit www.mlanet.org/resources/medspeak.) If you ask your doctor's office to call in a prescription, the nurse may need to check with the doctor, adding an extra step.

Let's say you go the pharmacy to pick up your prescription at 5:00 p.m. on a weekday. Both the pharmacy counter and drive-through are jam-packed. All of the pharmacists and pharmacy technicians are scrambling to get the right medication into the right bottles and then into the right bags with the right labels for the right customers. After you have purchased your medication, you take it home and follow the instructions carefully—or do you?

With all of these steps, it's a wonder we don't have a higher incidence of medication errors. Any broken link in the chain can yield devastating results. Potential causes for dangerous missteps include look-alike medicines; sound-alike medicines; interactions with other pharmaceutical drugs, herbal medications, homeopathic remedies, nutritional supplements, and over-the-counter drugs; miscommunication between physician and pharmacy, miscommunication between physician and patient about instructions, mix-ups with other customers at the pharmacy; medication side effects; and drug allergies, to name just a few.

Helping Yourself

Your most powerful weapon in reducing vulnerability to medication errors is your relationship with your pharmacist. Your pharmacist can spend more time with you than your physicians can, unless you seek the pharmacist's help during peak hours. He is more familiar with over-the-counter medications than your physician is. He can help you find safe ways to cut prescription costs and may contact your physician to request a generic alternative. In 22 states, pharmacists can prescribe nonnarcotic drugs and, with the proper certification, administer immunizations such as flu and shingles shots. Your pharmacist has broad-spectrum knowledge about disease states and medications, not to mention valuable insight on dosing instructions and dangerous interactions.

Tools for Tracking Your Medication

In addition to the medication spreadsheet recommended in chapter 4, you can also find tools online to help you keep track of medications and dosages. Visit www.jointcommission.org/PatientSafety/SpeakUp and select the brochure "Help Avoid Mistakes with Your Medicine" to find general medication safety information as well as a convenient wallet card for important contact information and a list of your medications.

The Vial of Life project (www.vialoflife.com) offers an online form you can use to record all of your vital health information, including medications. This program recommends putting the form in a resealable bag with other lifesaving information and keeping it taped to the refrigerator. Vial of Life provides decals to keep on the refrigerator, on the front door, and on your car.

Because senior citizens often take ten or more medications at a time, some senior centers have medical personnel available to help check for dangerous interactions and to make sure their clients are taking their medications properly. Our local senior center has a periodic brown-bag day and encourages seniors to bring in all medications, supplements, alternative treatments, and over-the-counter medications so that on-site nurses can do a safety check.

One pharmacy should be the central location of all of your medication information. If it is not, you need to transfer all your prescriptions to one pharmacy to reduce the risk of dangerous drug interactions. A pharmacy with a sophisticated computer system can flag dangerous interactions between different medications, but this is helpful only if you use just one pharmacy. This capability is especially critical if you are taking medications prescribed by different physicians.

To do your part in preventing dangerous drug interactions, you must, at a minimum, provide your PCP and your pharmacist with a list of all medications, herbal or homeopathic remedies, supplements, and over-the-counter medications you are taking. For further medication safety, take an updated medication list with you whenever you see a specialist, chiropractor, alternative practitioner, nutritionist, optometrist, or dentist.

For checks and balances, you can also search for drug-to-drug, drug-to-herbals-and-supplements, and drug-to-food interactions. An excellent resource is *The AARP Guide to Pills* by MaryAnne Hochadel, PharmD, BCPS. This book covers all of the interactions mentioned above and even the effects of some medications on medical tests. You can also search for a supplement or an herbal treatment individually at www.nlm.nih.gov/medlineplus/druginformation.html to screen for interactions with pharmaceutical drugs.

Safe Medication Practices

Perhaps your best line of defense is to read carefully the package insert that comes with your prescription for instructions on medications, supplements, and foods to avoid while taking the drug. After you read the insert, be sure to discard it in a shredder to reduce your vulnerability to identity theft. Most inserts include personal information such as date of birth, address, telephone number, and prescription number. If the insert does not include complete information on interactions, you can visit the medication manufacturer's Web site, or you can check the comprehensive drug index section at the Food and Drug Administration's site at www.fda.gov/cder/drug/DrugSafety/DrugIndex.htm.

Package inserts and the FDA's Web site both offer comprehensive information about medications, including risks and side effects. The Medline Plus site listed in the preceding paragraph also has a tool for looking up medications by name and reviewing crucial information. Peer-reviewed journals such as the *Journal of the American Medical Association*, *PubMed*, and the *New England Journal of Medicine* provide valuable information from the perspective of medical practitioners. You must educate yourself about the possible risks of any medication you take before you ingest it in any form, and weigh the benefit-to-risk ratio. Although you should consider the advice of your physician carefully, the final decision is yours.

The Institute for Safe Medicine Practices provides general information on medication safety at www.ismp.org. Its "Do Not Crush" list is a particularly useful feature since some medications are very unsafe when crushed or even split. Pill-splitting has become a symptom of our economy and the cost of medications, which are marked up as much as 800 percent. In the practice of pill-splitting, physicians write prescriptions for twice the recommended dosage so that patients can purchase the larger dosage for slightly more money but make the medicine last twice as long. This is a great way to save money, if done safely. The problem is that you cannot safely divide some medications, such as capsules, timed-release or enteric-coated medications, and others. Before you consider pill-splitting, check with both your physician and your pharmacist and buy a pill splitter so you can do it as safely as possible. Do not split an entire bottle of pills all at once. Some medications lose their efficacy when exposed to air for extended periods of time.

Additional safe medication practices include...

- *Selecting a physician who uses electronic medical records.* This is more easily said than done because this kind of records system is cost prohibitive for most physicians. However, an electronic system reduces the risk of medication errors by flagging potentially dangerous interactions.

- *Resisting the temptation to order medications online.* These medications are not regulated and may be counterfeit or, even worse, may contain dangerous ingredients not listed in the packaging. Medications from Canada are not regulated and are often manufactured in the US and China.

- *Checking your prescription bag before you leave the pharmacy* to ensure the medication label is correct and lists the correct dosage. As an added precaution, check the pills inside the bottles, and if they look different than you expect them to, ask the pharmacist about the difference. Most pharmacy errors occur because of customer bag mix-ups, but some are caused by look-alike and sound-alike medications. Be clear on the name and spelling of your medication. For more information on look-alike sound-alike medications, you can visit www.usp.org/hqi/similarProducts/drugErrorFinderTool.html to find drug names that have been associated with medication errors.

- *Following the dosing instructions exactly and contacting your physician or pharmacist with questions.* If you take several medications, you may need a pill organizer to stay on the proper dosing schedule. Whatever you do, don't stop a medication abruptly, unless directed by your physician. Some medications, such as prednisone and tricyclic antidepressants require tapering off to stop taking them safely.

- *Not sharing medications or taking others' medications.* This is unsafe and often inefficient. For example, if you take a friend's leftover antibiotics, you may feel better for a few days, but the symptoms will return if you don't take the full round of antibiotics to kill the infection.

- *Reporting any adverse effects from medications.* If you suffer a side effect listed in the insert, ask your physician to adjust your dosage or select another medication. If your adverse effect is not listed online or in the insert, you have an obligation to yourself and others to report it to the FDA through its Web site or by calling 1-800-FDA-1088.

Health Screening

Another proactive measure you can take is in the area of health screenings. Chapter 4 covers this topic briefly as an important patient responsibility. You cannot depend on your busy physician to let you know when it is time for an important screening. Even if your physician has an electronic system to alert him, the ultimate responsibility is yours. Testing can fall through the cracks easily when a physician has hundreds of patients.

Cancer is an insidious disease that is best prevented, if prevention is possible. The next best thing is early detection, which can make the difference between life and death. Cancer is expected to be the top killer by 2010 according to the World Health Organization, so we must be proactive in early detection efforts. The U.S. Preventive Services Task Force provides screening guidelines for major disease, including cancer, at www.ahrq.gov/clinic/pocketgd08. The American Cancer Society also offers screening guidelines and risk factors, including environmental toxins at www.cancer.org. You can also visit the National Cancer Institute's Web site at www.cancer.gov and review information from the American Society of Clinical Oncology at www.cancer.net.

One of the most important cancer screenings—though most often delayed due to its unpleasantness—is the colonoscopy. Gastroenterologist Dino Ferrante, MD, has diagnosed a number of patients with early-stage colon cancer through routine colonoscopies. These patients were proactive with their screenings and caught the cancer in a much more treatable stage. Dr. Ferrante recommends colonoscopies for healthy individuals with no symptoms starting at age 50.

Heart disease is another major killer. One of the best preventive measures you can take is regular blood pressure readings. Blood pressure increases with age and is a strong risk factor for heart disease. You can and should measure your blood pressure on a regular basis, especially if your systolic number is over 120 and your diastolic number is over 80. Another simple, but significant screening tool is regular cholesterol testing. Both the U.S. Preventive Services Task Force and the American Heart Association (www.americanheart.org) provide screening guidelines for cardiovascular diseases. The AHA also provides information on warning signs and a number of preventive tools.

For overall health screening and risk assessment information, check out familydoctor.org or www.mayoclinic.com/health/health-screening/WO00112. If you have an opportunity to attend a health fair, by all means please do so. Health fairs often offer vital services that include blood testing and screening for diseases and conditions such as breast cancer, prostate cancer, cardiovascular diseases, diabetes, osteoporosis, glaucoma, and mental health problems. These services are usually free or very low cost.

Working with Your Own Doctor

Perhaps your best defense is regular communication with your PCP. When asked which screenings are most critical, 58 percent of the respondents to the Physician Survey chose "Periodic Health Exams," 24 percent selected "Cardiovascular Screenings," and 16 percent chose "Cancer Screenings." One respondent brought up the excellent point that risk factors should guide physicians and patients in selecting important screenings, a sentiment echoed by professor of preventive medicine Daniel Blumenthal, MD, MPH. Dr. Blumenthal also encourages patients to report any changes in health status as soon as possible.

You and your PCP should discuss your risk factors for certain diseases regularly and stay current with their screenings. For example, if you smoke and have high blood pressure, you need regular cardiovascular and cancer screenings. If you are taking synthetic estrogen but not progesterone and still have your uterus, you have an increased risk of both breast cancer and cervical cancer. If you are taking an oral bisphosphonate for osteoporosis, be aware that you are at risk for esophagitis (inflammation of the tube leading to the stomach), particularly if you do not take the drug as directed. As reported to the U.S. Food and Drug Administration, in 54 esophageal cancer cases in the U.S., Canada, Europe, Australia, and Japan, an oral bisphosphonate was identified as either a suspect drug (48 cases) or concomitant drug (6 cases) (Wysowski, 2009). More patients who developed esophageal cancer with oral bisphosphonate use, including my mother, have been reported since the article was published.

Specialty Testing

If you have risk factors for a particular cancer, or any disease for that matter, you may benefit from a consultation with a geneticist. Your genetic structure may reveal your chances of getting cancer or another catastrophic illness. This emerging field, known as personalized medicine, will determine our risk for certain diseases based on our DNA and identify which specific treatment is needed.

When I asked Chris Gunter, PhD, director of research affairs at HudsonAlpha Institute of Biotechnology, how far we are from personalized medicine, she smiled and said, "We're already there." Dr. Gunter pointed out that breast cancer, for example, is not just one disease. It is at least six different diseases, and careful study of a patient's DNA or cells can already identify some specific ones. Once a doctor identifies the type of cancer, she can administer the appropriate treatment. This type of research led to the discovery of the breast cancer drug Herceptin by oncologist and researcher Dennis Slamon, MD, PhD.

Genetic testing is already available for breast and ovarian cancers through study of the BRCA1 and BRCA2 genes. Alterations in these genes indicate a vulnerability to breast or ovarian cancer. Keep in mind that 90 percent of these cancers are not inherited. In weighing the risks and benefits of this kind of testing, be mindful of all of your risk factors, including prior cancer history, family history, hormone replacement therapy, alcohol and tobacco use, unhealthy diet, and lack of exercise. If you have a number of risk factors, you may benefit from testing.

After meeting with Dr. Gunter, I have a better understanding of the difference between genetics and genomics, primarily one of scale. The study of genetics is directed at DNA and evaluates one gene at a time. We have about 20,000 genes in our genetic code of about three billion letters. Genomics looks at the entire gene makeup of the human body at once, and in 2009, we can sequence the three billion letters in our genetic code in a month. HudsonAlpha is participating in The Cancer Genome Atlas (TCGA), a National Institutes of Health–sponsored program designed to create an atlas of genomic changes that lead to cancer. TCGA addresses three types of cancer—brain, lung, and ovarian—and its goals are to target the best treatments and clinical trials for each patient, discover risk factors, and develop prevention strategies. To learn more about this project, visit http://cancergenome.nih.gov/.

Not all diseases are inherited, but researchers have identified cancer as genetic, meaning cancer is caused by mutations from DNA. Other complex genetic diseases include Parkinson's disease, cystic fibrosis, Crohn's disease, diabetes, and arthritis. HudsonAlpha is currently studying a number of these by looking at large groups of patients vs. non-affected individuals and comparing the letters in their genetic codes. Toxicogenomics is a subspecialty that examines the effect that toxins (environmental and dietary) have on the body and on a person's susceptibility to these effects based on DNA, and HudsonAlpha researchers will soon begin studies in the area as well. The study of genetics and genomics is still young, but researchers have made a great deal of progress.

Trust Your Intuition Too

Screening and high-tech testing are very important in disease prevention and early detection, but I have to put in a plug for good, old-fashioned intuition. A mother's intuition is exceptionally powerful. Thirteen years ago, Taylor noticed that her 11-day-old son, Grant, was in trouble. He had a fever and jaundice, and he refused to nurse. Taylor called the pediatrician's office repeatedly, only to be treated like a hysterical mother (Grant is her third child) and told, "It's nothing. He'll be fine."

Her intuition told her otherwise, and she took Grant to the emergency room, where a team of eight doctors and nurses quickly gathered around Grant's bed and began testing and treatment. The ER staff discovered a piece of tissue on his ureter that was causing urine to back up into his kidneys, a condition that would have been fatal if left untreated. Grant had emergency surgery to remove the tissue, and today, thanks to his mother's intuition and the ER staff, he is a thriving 13-year-old who recently performed a lead role in a local production of Les Misérables.

Wellness and prevention require effort and commitment, as you can see. When I met with Lennox Marr, oncology nurse manager, I asked him for his opinion on the ratio of responsibility between the patient and the medical profession. He believes that 90 percent of the responsibility for health care falls on the patient and 10 percent rests with the medical profession.

From all that I have learned through my own experiences and while conducting research for this book, I wholeheartedly agree with his assessment. With dwindling health-care resources, now more than ever, patients must step up and assume responsibility.

Chapter 4

The Rights and Responsibilities of Patients

Proactively Using Health Care

The previous two chapters offered wellness and prevention initiatives as ways to assume personal health-care responsibility. These are great basics, but there are plenty of additional ways to take ownership of your health care. Although medical practitioners are an important part of your team, you are ultimately in charge. If your health-care team and support system were a large company, you would be the CEO. And yes, you can hire and fire at will. If one physician cannot help you, there is no reason why you cannot find another with whom you are comfortable. I hope you do not have to hire 38 doctors to find the right diagnosis like I did, but you must do whatever is necessary to get the help you need. The point is, you have the right to seek the best medical care possible.

Patients' rights have been a hot topic in recent years. In 1998, the President's Advisory Commission on Consumer Protection and Quality in the Health Care Industry issued its final report, which included the Consumer Bill of Rights and Responsibilities (President's Advisory Commission 1998). In 2001, Senators McCain, Edwards, and Kennedy introduced the Bipartisan Patient Protection Act, S 1052, offering more freedoms to patients in the areas of health-care coverage and clinical trials. A number of medical institutions and state governments also publish patient bills of rights and responsibilities, indicating the need for equal participation from patients. As a patient, you have both the right and the responsibility to participate in your diagnosis and treatment.

After much reflection on these various bills of rights and responsibilities and on my own journey, I created the Proactive Patient Bill of Rights and the Proactive Patient Bill of Responsibilities. These principles are key in helping you navigate the health-care system and gain full advantage from it. Remember—you are in charge!

The Proactive Patient Bill of Rights

The right to equal participation in your medical care. You have the right to participate equally in deciding which tests and treatments will be used in your care. You have the right to ask questions, share your own research, and request any reasonable tests or treatments. You also have the right to refuse any tests or treatments that are risky, painful, cost prohibitive, or in direct violation of your religious beliefs.

The right to information about diagnosis, planned treatment, alternate treatments, risks, and prognosis. You have the legal and ethical right to give informed consent to treatments and procedures. Medical practitioners are required to obtain your written authorization prior to certain procedures and treatments. You do not have to grant this authorization until you have been informed fully about all aspects of the treatment or procedure, including benefits, risks, the reason for the treatment or procedure, any alternatives available and their benefits and risks, and the consequences of choosing not to authorize the treatment or procedure. If you are physically unable to grant authorization, you may appoint a trusted friend or family member to do it for you.

For treatment and procedures offering little or no risk, your physician or nurse needs only simple consent rather than the more formal informed consent in writing. These procedures include blood tests, medication prescriptions, and referrals to specialists. You can authorize simple consent by following through with the practitioner's recommendation.

The right to know the name, role, and credentials of each health-care provider responsible for your care. You can ask for this information directly from the provider or from the health-care facility. Chapter 5 provides detailed definitions of the initials after your health-care provider's name. You can check out physicians' credentials online by visiting www .ama-assn.org/ama/pub/patients/patients.shtml and clicking on Doctor Finder. You can find physicians' credentials and patients' ratings at www.healthgrades.com and www.aarp.org/health/doctors. You can view hospital ratings at www.healthgrades.com and www.leapfrog group.org/for_consumers.

The right to information on clinical trials for which you may be eligible. Although you have this right, be mindful of your doctor's patient load and her ability to keep up with the latest trials. No doctor can be expected to keep up with all trials for all conditions under her purview. You may need to do a large part of the research for a specific condition. To gather information on federally funded trials, you can visit clinicaltrials .gov. For information on cancer trials, you can search www.cancer.gov/ clinicaltrials or go to www.cancer.net and click on Clinical Trials.

The right to prompt emergency care without prior authorization or financial consideration. The Emergency Medical Treatment and Active Labor Act (EMTALA) of 1986 (informally called the patient antidumping law) requires hospitals and ambulance services to provide treatment to anyone needing emergency medical care. The EMTALA applies to Centers for Medicare and Medicaid Services (CMS) hospitals, or those that receive payment from Medicare or Medicaid. Because most hospitals accept Medicare and Medicaid, the EMTALA covers nearly all hospitals.

Any patient who visits the emergency department of a participating hospital must receive treatment regardless of insurance coverage or ability to pay. The hospital must provide a screening exam, treatment for and stabilization of the emergency medical condition, and, if necessary, transfer of the stabilized patient to a facility with greater capabilities for treatment. No patient can be discharged without proper treatment. Hospitals that violate the EMTALA face stiff penalties (American Academy of Emergency Medicine 2009).

The right to be treated respectfully and without discrimination. Your medical providers must treat you respectfully without regard to gender, race, religion, national origin, disability, or sexual orientation. They do not have the right to subject you to sexual harassment, which is unwelcome behavior of a sexual nature. Sexual behavior is sometimes difficult to define within the parameters of medical care. Your provider has to be up close and personal with you in order to get the job done. Your role is to determine what is and is not appropriate to that situation. If you consult a doctor for abdominal pain and he massages your shoulders, tries to hug you tightly, and removes your gown to use a stethoscope (this happened to me), his behavior is inappropriate. When in doubt, listen to your gut. If you encounter a doctor who is clearly behaving badly, contact your state medical board.

The right to confidentiality and privacy. For more information on your rights under the Health Insurance Portability and Accountability Act (HIPAA), visit the Office for Civil Rights at www.hhs.gov/ocr/hipaa. This site provides extensive information on your right to privacy with your health information. Your health providers must keep all medical records, as well as discussions regarding your medical care, private and confidential.

The right to access your medical records. You have a legal right to all medical documents that pertain to you. Although you have to nearly sign your life away to authorize anyone else to see them under HIPAA, you do have the right to copies of your own records. You have the right to see what is in every medical report and what each provider has said about your case. But be careful what you wish for. This is how I found out that I'm suffering from conflict about my role as a Southern woman!

The right to a second or even third opinion. You have the right to double-check any diagnosis that seems erroneous or that subjects you to painful or risky treatments. Research shows that getting a second opinion results in a new diagnosis in as many as 30 percent of cases (Klitzman

2008). A second opinion is a must if you are diagnosed with a life-threatening illness or advised to undergo surgery. If your health-care network refuses to pay for a second or third opinion, don't be afraid to use the appeal process. The more you appeal and the further you go up the chain of command, the more likely you are to get your insurance provider to pay for that additional consultation.

The right to a reasonable choice of providers. Your plan should provide you with high-quality health care as needed. You have the right to know all the options under your plan, and you have probably received a booklet with that information from your insurance provider. If not, you can call the phone number on your insurance card or check your provider's Web site for the information. If your coverage is part of a group plan provided by your employer, your company benefits administrator can be a great source of help.

The right to an interpreter for hearing-impaired patients or people who do not speak English. Health-care facilities must make a reasonable effort to provide interpreters for those who need them. Communication between doctors and patients is difficult enough without a language barrier.

The right to request and receive a reasonable estimate of charges for medical care. This is particularly crucial for any charges medical insurance does not cover. Unfortunately, we have to look at cost as a factor when making decisions about our health care.

The right to receive a copy of an itemized bill for services. You may be surprised at what you find on a hospital bill. Some hospitals overcharge patients with health insurance to recover their losses on those without it. This practice is known as cost shifting. You have the right to question any charges that look suspicious, particularly if your insurance plan will not cover them.

The right to appeal or file a grievance with a health-care provider or facility, a medical insurance provider, or the appropriate state licensing agency for any violation of your rights as a patient. You have the right to know all procedures for filing a complaint with any provider or medical facility. Most insurance providers and medical facilities provide written guidelines for filing complaints. If not, you have the right to ask for them. And remember, the higher you ascend the chain of command, the better the chances of successfully resolving your concerns.

Patient rights and responsibilities are interrelated. If you have a particular right, then you also have responsibility for assuming that right. I cover most of these topics in more detail in later chapters, offering specific tools for assuming the responsibilities.

The Proactive Patient Bill of Responsibilities

Take your health seriously. If you don't take your health seriously, neither will your doctor. Your doctor cannot help you unless you are putting forth the effort to maintain overall wellness. If you are not living a healthy lifestyle, your body cannot heal. Your diabetes medication is only a Band-Aid approach if you are not following a healthy diet. If you have a heart condition, your doctor cannot help you if you maintain a high-fat diet and use tobacco products. Your desire for good health must outweigh your need for unhealthy habits.

Be vigilant about getting regular screening tests. You are responsible for knowing which screenings you need and when, based on age, family history, and risk factors. To find a list of recommended screenings by age, check out Web MD: women.webmd.com/tc/early-disease -detection-overview. Although these recommendations appear in the women's section of the site, the listing includes men's screenings, such as prostate and testicular cancer. So, guys, you're not off the hook!

Find the best primary-care physician possible. In most cases, your primary-care physician will be a family practitioner or an internist. Your PCP will be a generalist and the focal point of all your medical care, referring to you appropriate specialists as needed and intervening on your behalf for emergency medical care. In addition to checking the credentials and any past or pending disciplinary action of your PCP, you also need to ensure that she has hospital privileges. If you need to visit the emergency department or stay in the hospital, you will need a PCP with privileges at that hospital to coordinate treatment with the emergency department or to oversee your treatment in the hospital.

Coordinate your care from several different medical practitioners. To ensure that you are not receiving treatments that conflict with one another, make sure your PCP knows about medical care you are receiving from any specialists you have found on your own or from alternative practitioners. You may find that one doctor needs to share your records and, in some cases, X-ray films with other doctors. It is your responsibility to follow up to make sure this happens, even if it means hand delivering reports and films yourself. You must also be the focal point when you have several medical practitioners working together on your case. You cannot assume that all of your doctors are communicating effectively with one another.

Disclose fully all health-related information with all your medical practitioners, even if it means disclosing something unflattering or embarrassing that you would rather not reveal. If you have a poor diet or a history of mental illness, substance abuse, or unprotected sex or you just can't seem to break that nicotine or caffeine addiction, your doctor needs to know. You must also apprise him of all family medical history. A number of serious diseases are hereditary, and your doctor cannot be alert to your risk without full knowledge of your family history. He must have all the pieces in order to solve the puzzle, and this includes your emotional and spiritual well-being. You may find that he is interested in knowing about nonmedical aspects of your life such as family, work, and hobbies. In recent years, the medical community has gotten more involved in treating the whole person rather than just the physical symptoms. If your doctor seems nosy, be grateful— you are receiving holistic care.

Keep in mind that respect is a two-way street. I reviewed the responses to the Physician Survey question regarding patient etiquette and found many of the responses appalling. Physicians reported inappropriate patient behavior ranging from texting and talking on cell phones during office visits to physical assaults in the emergency department. The more respect you show for your medical providers and the time that you spend together, the more you are likely to get in return. You are responsible for keeping appointments and, when you are unable to do so, to make every effort to cancel at least 24 hours in advance. Eliminate distractions to the best of your ability during your consultations. Remember, you will probably have no more than ten minutes to present your case and get the help you need. And yes, this means turning off your cell phone!

Help your doctor help you. Ask thought-provoking questions to help your doctor expand the possibilities. If you are having trouble finding the right diagnosis, ask questions such as, "What else could it be?" or, "Which parts of the body are near the source of my symptoms?" Clarify any confusion or misunderstanding you have about anything your doctor has said during the consultation, even if it means calling his office later. You should also provide feedback to let your doctor know whether or not a possible treatment is helping your symptoms. This not only helps him narrow down your case, but your feedback may help with future patients. Doctors and nurses want and need to know when they have helped a patient. They entered this helping profession for a reason.

Recognize the human fallibility of health-care professionals. Although medical practitioners and facilities are cognizant of their own fallibility and employ a number of safeguards, errors may still occur. This is where you come in. Speak up and question anything that looks or sounds suspicious. Make sure you have a trusted advocate with you when you are hospitalized or need emergency care. Request copies of all diagnostic and screening tests and double-check the results. Research possible diagnoses and treatments on your own and present the information to your doctor.

Be aware that your PCP knows a little bit about a lot of different medical issues and has to look at what is going on throughout your entire body. If you suspect a problem in a particular area of the body, don't be shy about asking to see a specialist. Keep in mind that although your PCP should be on the lookout for various cancers, she may not make the connection between symptoms and a possible cancer threat. If you have any reason to suspect cancer, don't wait for your doctor to broach the subject. Be proactive and insist on the appropriate diagnostic tests.

Follow your doctor's instructions cooperatively. Forty percent of the time, a disease's worsening is caused by the patient's noncompliance with medical advice. You are responsible for taking medication as directed; following instructions for lab work, X-rays, and invasive testing procedures carefully; and complying with any treatment recommended by your physician, such as physical therapy. Speak up if the doctor suggests something you don't think you can pursue or maintain. Be sure you understand all aspects of your protocol, contacting your doctor's office as often as necessary.

Participate actively in your diagnosis and treatment. Don't sit back and let your doctor make all the decisions for your care. Take ownership. You are responsible for your decisions, so you must be as well informed as possible. Ask your doctor for detailed information about recommended tests and treatments. Be proactive, and keep up with all tests results, treatments, and referrals. Be the squeaky wheel that gets the grease if you are experiencing any delays in diagnosis or treatment. Your doctor's office may not call to inform you of test results, so be prepared to call and get that information.

Arm yourself with as much information as possible. Your primary-care physician cannot possibly know everything about every medical condition. If you are referred to a specialist, you will learn more about a specific condition, but you may need to find additional information on your own. You can find an infinite amount of medical information online, but your challenge is determining which sites are reliable and which are not. "Into the Abyss" offers strategies for finding reputable sites, and the Resources at a Glance section in the back of the book includes a complete listing of recommended sites.

Medical Web Sites for Patient Empowerment

For additional guidelines you can visit www.nlm.nih.gov/medlineplus/healthywebsurfing.html. The Joint Commission, the accrediting body that helps health care organizations help patients through the provision of health care accreditation and related services that support performance improvement, offers a plethora of patient empowerment tools at www.jointcommission.org/GeneralPublic and at www.joint commission.org/PatientSafety/SpeakUp. The Agency for Healthcare Research and Quality provides information on topics such as wellness and prevention, health plans, and surgical and medication safety at www.ahrq.gov/consumer. The American College of Surgeons also offers a number of patient resources at www.facs.org/patienteducation. Additional reputable sites include www.webmd.com, health.discovery .com, www.mayoclinic.com, and www.pubmed.com.

Manage your medications. Use just one pharmacy to avoid dangerous drug interactions. You must have one central source for your medications; there is too much room for error with more than one. Most pharmacies have sophisticated computer systems that flag dangerous interactions. But as an added precaution, you should check medications before you take them to make sure you received the correct prescription. Learn as much about medications' side effects and interactions as possible. Talk to your pharmacist, look at the package inserts, check the Web sites of the drug manufacturers, and check online for postings from patients who have experienced troubling side effects.

Call in refills on your medications several days before you run out in case the pharmacy has to order more. If you use a national pharmacy chain, you may be able to get your medication at another of the chain's stores in town if your regular store does not have it in stock.

If you call your doctor's office for more refills, be sure to do it well before you run out of your medication, and have your pharmacy's phone number ready to give your doctor's office staff.

Know your medical-insurance plan. It is your responsibility to know how your medical group or HMO works, which health-care professionals are covered, and what to do after office hours. You need to know which precertification rules apply to various medical procedures. If you do not have this information, make sure you get it by calling your provider, checking its Web site, or contacting your company's benefits administrator. If you have Medicare or Medicaid, you do not have to stay within a network, but some physicians and facilities do not accept Medicare or Medicaid patients. It is your responsibility to find out where you can receive care. To find out which physicians and facilities accept Medicare or Medicaid patients, you can call the local medical society or association.

Manage your medical records even if all is well. If nothing else, you get to find out what your doctors think of you. I learned that not only was I suffering from conflict about my role as a Southern woman, I was also depressed, anxious, obsessive-compulsive, suffering from an organic mood disorder, overweight, and not very smart. Unflattering labels aside, you need to know which tests and evaluations are normal so that you can have a baseline. You can obtain copies of most of your records from your primary care physician. Your file will probably contain reports for office visits with your PCP and with specialists recommended by your PCP, as well as lab work, X-rays, diagnostic procedures, surgical procedures, and hospital summary reports. If your PCP does not have any of these reports, you need to contact the specialist, lab, imaging center, or hospital directly.

You may have to pay for copies of your records, but the expense is well worth it. The more familiar you are with your history, the more efficiently you can work with your medical practitioners. You cannot count on your PCP to keep up with your history, which tests you've had, which medications you are taking, and so on. Remember, he is seeing 25 to 50 patients per day, and your specialists are even less familiar with your medical history.

Comply with all health-care facility rules and regulations affecting patient care and conduct. Rules and regulations are necessary for the safety, comfort, and quality care of all patients, particularly during hospital stays. You may not like or even understand some of the regulations, but they exist for a reason.

Fulfill your financial obligations as promptly as possible. Medical expenses can escalate quickly, and you may not be able to pay your out-of-pocket expenses. Most medical facilities will work with you to create a fair and reasonable payment plan. If you find yourself in this situation, you need at least one ally in the accounting or finance department.

Prepare thoroughly for all consultations. This topic is extensive and significant enough to require its own large discussion section below. Keep in mind that the average internist must see 25 patients per day to make ends meet. The average family practitioner sees about 50 patients per day. Your time with your doctor is extremely limited, so you must take advantage of every second.

Preparing for Consultations

Throughout my lengthy medical journey, I approached each visit with a new doctor as I would a college exam or a job interview. It made sense to go about something as important as an undiagnosed, disabling medical condition with at least as much care. I prepared background information days or weeks in advance, making sure all documents were updated and sometimes even sending information to the doctor ahead of time.

I developed a number of tools that were helpful in my pursuit of a diagnosis and treatment. These tools and their applications are described at the end of this chapter, and they are available for download at www.theproactivepatient.com. The Resources at a Glance section in the back of the book also includes sample forms.

These tools are helpful for an office visit or even for a scheduled hospitalization. But what if you require a sudden trip to the emergency room? The beauty of the system is that most of your history is within reach and reasonably up to date on your computer. Keep in mind that emergency room doctors don't have the benefit of your medical history, and this could hinder their ability to provide optimal care. You must provide as much information as quickly as possible, when you are least able to do so. With your health information easily accessible, you can quickly print out your list of medications, along with your lists of previous surgeries and hospitalizations, chronic conditions, and, if possible, a diary of your urgent symptoms.

If you want to carry convenience a step further, consider putting your medical history online so that it is just a couple of mouse clicks away from any practitioners whom you authorize to access your records. Several sites, such as www.passportmd.com, www.google.com/health, and www.safemedicaldata.com offer this service. Before you send your medical history out into cyberspace, read the site's information carefully to determine how much security and privacy are offered. Make sure the site is in compliance with HIPAA laws and that it will encrypt your information for safety. Look for sites that begin with "https" rather than "http." The "s" indicates that the site is secure.

All of these patient responsibilities may seem daunting. Yes, it takes a lot of effort to be a proactive patient. As CEO of your body, you are responsible for the oversight associated with your health care. But your medical care is like anything else in life. The more effort you put into it, the greater the rewards you will reap. As Mom often said, God helps those who help themselves.

Helpful Tools for Diagnosis and Treatment Consultations

1. *Question list.* A question list is a godsend during an office visit. You may be nervous, desperate, or rushed. You might forget important points or questions. If your entire future hinges on this particular doctor's ability and willingness to find the answer, you may be intimidated

or emotional. If you develop a list of questions ahead of time, you won't be as likely to forget something important, and you can make better use of those few precious minutes.

The nature of your questions will depend on where you are in the diagnostic process, whether or not your condition is chronic, your history with this physician, and a number of other factors. You will need basic information from your doctor such as office policies and procedures, how test results are communicated, and why medications are prescribed and which side effects you might experience. Depending on your doctor's preference, you might need to bring two copies of your question list. Some doctors prefer to review the question list before they enter the exam room; others prefer to hear the questions directly from the patient. The nurse will have a good idea of the doctor's preference.

2. *Symptom list.* Keep your symptom list updated, adding new symptoms as they appear. When describing your symptoms, be as specific as possible. Keep in mind that the doctor cannot feel what you're feeling. Aim to let her do that with your description of your symptoms. If your symptoms have not changed since your last visit with that doctor, this list is not necessary since your current list should be in your chart.

3. *Diary, journal, or chronology of symptoms.* Start tracking your symptoms from the beginning, and add entries as you see changes or further deterioration. Keep a detailed record of what makes the symptoms better or worse. If you have attempted any treatments, keep a journal of what effects, if any, they have had on your symptoms. This document will become lengthy if you have tried a number of treatments and have experienced the symptoms for a long time. But that is okay; a caring doctor will want to know your history. If you have ongoing visits with your doctor, you need to provide her with ongoing updates. You should bring two copies of your updated list to each office visit so that you and your doctor can review the list simultaneously while discussing what has transpired since your last visit.

4. *Research items.* If you have found information on the Internet that

you think might be helpful to your case, organize it for quick scanning and bring it to your appointment. If your doctor is threatened by this, you will know very quickly that you need to find another doctor. It's better to realize this sooner than later.

5. *Current medications and drug allergies.* I recommend this spreadsheet for anyone who consults a doctor at any time for any reason. How many times have you visited a new doctor only to be given the usual onslaught of questionnaires to complete? At least one form will ask for current medications and dosages. How are you supposed to remember which meds you take and at which dosages? It gets even more complicated if you also take supplements. And yes, they need to be included in your medication information as well. "Natural" does not always mean safe. Remember ephedra? The spreadsheet I keep has categories for daily medications, as-needed medications, and supplements. For each, I list the name, dosage, and reason I take it. Most medical questionnaires ask about drug allergies, but it doesn't hurt to have them listed on a spreadsheet as a precaution. You can't be too careful with something this serious.

6. *Past surgeries and hospitalizations.* Depending on the depth of your medical history, you may want to divide this document into two spreadsheets. Again, this tool is helpful for anyone who visits the doctor or emergency room at any time for any reason. You will be asked for this information on a questionnaire any time you visit a new doctor or medical facility. Wouldn't it be nice to just scribble in the space, "See attached"? You will need to include in your spreadsheet the when, where, and what for all your past surgeries and hospitalizations.

7. *Chronic medical conditions.* Your doctor needs to know about other chronic conditions for which you are being treated. This may seem like a small matter, but it can be huge. For example, if I seek treatment for a bacterial infection, the doctor needs to know that I have ulcerative colitis, which is greatly aggravated by certain antibiotics. The column headings I use for the chronic conditions sheet include Condition, Positive Test Result, Doctor Treating the Condition, and

Treatment Status. This information gives credibility to your medical history and will make a doctor less likely to wonder, "Does she really have all these things wrong with her?"

8. *Attempted treatments.* If you have tried numerous treatments for a specific condition, your condition may warrant its own spreadsheet. I ended up with a three-page spreadsheet that lists the attempted treatment, the type of treatment, when it was attempted, and the results. This method helps the doctor scan the information quickly to figure out what to try next.

9. *Tests.* I hope and pray you don't end up with a three-page spread-sheet like I did. I have endured a lot of testing. My spreadsheet has three columns: Test Performed, Date, and Results. Doctors find this more expeditious than pouring through a mountain of test reports.

10. *Medical-records binder.* This tool has been a double-edged sword for me. Many doctors find all this information helpful, but some find it threatening. One doctor even threw my binder across the room! My stack of reports from various medical facilities had become so huge that I bought a three-inch binder to hold them. I decided it would be easier for doctors to scan the various reports quickly if I divided the information by medical facility, and each facility visit has its own neon page divider. For example, the reports from my visit to the Mayo Clinic are preceded by a bright pink sheet with the name of the facility, the dates, the physicians I consulted, and the tests that were done.

Chapter 5

What Kind of Practitioner Do I Need?

Surveying Ability and Availability

As patients, we expect our practitioners to be superhuman as they work long hours diagnosing elusive conditions, selecting just the right treatment and dosage, or performing intricate surgery. We expect them to perform these tasks cheerfully, efficiently, and flawlessly. After all, we expect to get the most out of our expensive insurance coverage.

We envision our doctors going home from their offices to their mansions, where their paid domestic staffs have clean rooms, clean laundry, and nice dinners waiting. On weekends, they socialize with other doctors at the country club. Ah, what an idyllic life!

Not so fast! My collaboration with Dr. Wyatt and interviews with a number of primary-care physicians and specialists certainly helped me break through the mystique and dispelled some common misconceptions about the field of medicine. Physicians' lives are more difficult and less glamorous than they appear.

Imagine starting your work day at 6:30 a.m., seeing patients in the hospital after sleeping only two or three hours because you had an emergency hospital admission in the middle of the night. You race to make it to the office by 8:15 to start seeing patients there. Because you are a primary-care physician, you have to see a large number of patients to make ends meet. You see 15 during the morning, stopping only to meet with a drug rep who stops by, and then you have to take calls from other physicians. You have 25 minutes for lunch before you see another 15 patients during the afternoon while battling fatigue and drowsiness. You finally complete the patient visits and have a chance to catch up with paperwork around 5:30 p.m.

By 6:15 you head home, where you and your tired spouse negotiate who will watch the children and who will start dinner. Your spouse must also work full-time, because you are still paying off student loans, and with malpractice premiums and other overhead costs associated with your practice, money is tight. Throughout the evening, you are paged three times and must return calls and dispense medical advice via telephone. You would like to get online to look at some peer-reviewed journals to help you stay current in your field, but you are exhausted and collapse into bed by 10:00. You know you need to be at the hospital the next morning by 6:30, and you hope you can sleep through the night without receiving any emergency pages.

Not all physicians have such a demanding schedule, but some live the life described above. During my research, I uncovered a number of realities that dispel the following myths.

---

13 Myths About Doctors

Myth #1: Doctors go into medicine for the money or status. There are easier ways to obtain money and status, and they don't require 12 years of schooling. It takes much more than the prospect of wealth to endure the grueling training required to practice medicine.

Myth #2: All doctors are rich. It depends on the field of medicine. Certain specialties, such as neurosurgery, orthopedics, and cardiology command higher salaries and fees. Primary-care physicians, on the other hand, struggle to make ends meet, particularly in a solo practice. During lean months, they sometimes have to forego a salary to meet overhead. Malpractice insurance premiums have forced a number of doctors out of business.

Myth #3: Doctors are arrogant and condescending and have God complexes. As in any profession, some doctors are arrogant and others are very caring. What may seem like arrogance is often a standard for excellence as a result of 7 to 12 years of postgraduate schooling. The commitment to medical training is so enormous that physicians take pride in their accomplishments.

Myth #4: Doctors are insensitive. Doctors have to develop a thick skin in order to survive an emotionally wrenching career. If they get too emotionally involved, they lose their objectivity. They continually struggle to find the balance between art and science. Yes, they need to be caring, but their number one goal is diagnosis and treatment. Their time with patients is extremely limited, and circumstances force them to be constrained in interactions with their patients.

Myth #5: Doctors are happy to answer your medical questions when you run into them at the grocery store, drugstore, and so on. Discussing medical problems during your doctor's personal time is taboo unless you have an after-hours emergency and follow proper protocol. However, if you have a true emergency on a weekend, both you and your physician will be better off if you call the after-hours answering service and request a call from your doctor. Monday mornings are difficult enough, and if you wait until Monday morning to call with an emergency, your case will receive less attention.

Myth #6: A malpractice suit against a doctor is a red flag. The average surgeon is sued three times during his career. Keep in mind that anybody can sue for any reason at any time. A settlement offered by a physician is not always an admission of guilt, but often a way of settling the case quickly because his busy schedule does not allow for the court appearances and documentation associated with a lawsuit. Most physicians are aware of the constant threat of lawsuits and spend a lot of time on documentation that will protect them. Some admit to ordering tests that they don't believe are completely necessary just to protect themselves against the threat of litigation.

Myth #7: Careless doctors make mistakes. Human doctors make mistakes.

Nobody is perfect. Errors made by medical practitioners are very serious, and that is why the medical profession uses a larger number of safeguards than most professions. Physicians depend not only on support staff for checks and balances, but also on patients.

Myth #8: Medical practitioners are very healthy. Hospital nurses suffer more back injuries than any other profession because of the excessive lifting they must do. Doctors and support personnel are often less healthy than the general population because of exposure to contagious conditions. But doctors cannot just take sick days like other professions because even a one-day absence creates total chaos. You may not like the idea of your doctor's examining you while battling a cold or flu, but imagine how upset you would feel if her office called to cancel your appointment after you had carefully planned it around your work and family schedules.

Myth #9: Doctors remind you when you are due for screenings. Knowing when you are due for screenings is your responsibility. Unless your physician is part of a thriving group practice that can afford a $50,000 electronic medical-records system, she will not remember your screenings any more than she does those of her other 1500-plus patients.

Myth #10: Doctors welcome your Web-site research. It depends on where you get your research. If it is a forward from someone who heard it from her brother-in-law's sister's first cousin, your doctor is probably not interested. He will be much more receptive to a peer-reviewed article from *JAMA* or the *New England Journal of Medicine*.

Myth #11: Doctors all know each other—they have their own fraternity, they all socialize together, and so on. Unless your PCP has worked with a specialist, she probably doesn't know him nearly as well as you do. As for socializing, most physicians have very little time for a social life because of the demands of their profession.

Myth #12: All patients are treated equally regardless of insurance coverage.

"Good patient" is a code phrase that means the patient has good insurance coverage that pays well and quickly. Physicians need a high percentage of "good patients." This may sound cold, but everyone has to make a living, and slow, low-paying insurance negatively affects the lives of physicians. I spoke to a physician recently who suffered a $25,000 pay cut in 2008 because of delays in reimbursements. Physicians may also hesitate to recommend certain tests to patients with poor coverage.

Myth #13: Doctors are not interested in your personal life. A good doctor will treat the whole person and understand that mind and body are very much connected. A patient who is in chronic pain will probably suffer from depression. A patient without good emotional support may find healing more difficult than a patient with a healthy support system. When Dr. Wyatt trained residents, he quizzed them when they left a patient's hospital room, asking them to name three things they saw on the patient's nightstand. If a patient's nightstand only contained a water pitcher, telephone, and pen, this was an indication of a solitary existence and, probably, lack of a support system. A patient's nightstand with flowers and cards indicated a stronger support system.

As you can see, physicians must have a strong desire for such a daunting career path. They exhibit this passion from the very beginning because without a strong passion for medicine and for helping others, they cannot survive the demanding training. Dr. Wyatt's description of his arduous, sleep-deprived residency is a case in point. During his residency, he once worked 72 hours nonstop with no sleep. A study of residents in his program revealed that they were earning less than minimum wage when they divided their income by the number of hours worked. When I asked Dr. Wyatt if he ever wondered if all the sacrifice was worth it, he answered without hesitation, "Never." Clearly, the medical profession is not a career; it is a calling.

A Demanding Process

The chart on the following page illustrates the demanding educational requirements for a medical doctor. As you see, the progression is very lengthy. Many medical students do not make it through this process.

The first step in the process, undergraduate education, is the last opportunity the student will have for a normal life. As an undergraduate, she can still enjoy the college social experience somewhat, but she must keep her grades up to be competitive for a slot in her medical school program of choice. Medical schools accept students with varying academic backgrounds, but the most common undergraduate degrees are in chemistry, biology, physics, anatomy and physiology, and genetics.

Most premed students complete an undergraduate degree, although it is not required if all prerequisite coursework is completed. By junior year, the student needs to become serious about applying to medical schools and preparing for the Medical College Admission Test (MCAT). The MCAT is an exhausting five-hour test on physical sciences, verbal reasoning, writing, and biological sciences, and students can take it a maximum of three times per year. This gives them the opportunity to retake it in hopes of achieving a higher score. The higher the score, the better the chances of acceptance into the program of choice.

A medical school is part of an academic institution that teaches medicine. Acceptance into a medical school program is based on MCAT scores, grade point average, admissions essay, applicant interview, undergraduate research projects, and extracurricular and leadership activities. The standard medical school curriculum lasts four years, with two years of basic sciences and two years of clinical rotations, where students begin to work with patients. The rotations expose students to various fields of medicine to help them determine which one they would like to pursue upon completion of medical school.

Students who graduate from medical school receive an MD (medical doctor) or DO (doctor of osteopathy) degree. MD and DO training are very similar, and both degrees allow for licensing in all 50 states and hospital privileges. However, DOs focus on treating the patient as a whole, rather than on just one area of the body. They receive an additional 300 to 500 hours of training on the musculoskeletal system, and they offer

How a Doctor Becomes a Doctor

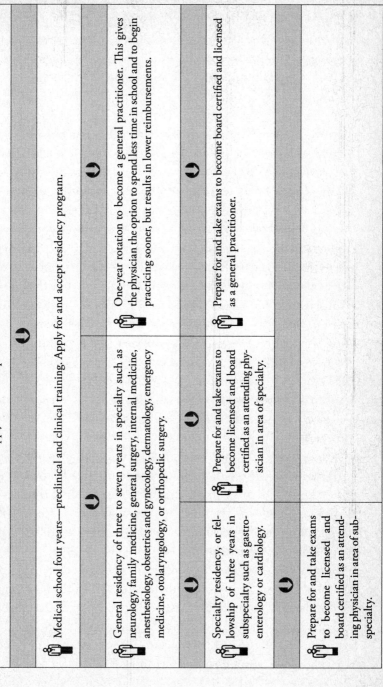

Earn a BS or BA degree in pre-med, biology, chemistry, physics, or related field, or complete prerequisite coursework. Prepare for and take MCAT exam for medical school admission. Apply for and accept medical school admission.

Medical school four years—preclinical and clinical training. Apply for and accept residency program.

General residency of three to seven years in specialty such as neurology, family medicine, general surgery, internal medicine, anesthesiology, obstetrics and gynecology, dermatology, emergency medicine, otolaryngology, or orthopedic surgery.

One-year rotation to become a general practitioner. This gives the physician the option to spend less time in school and to begin practicing sooner, but results in lower reimbursements.

Prepare for and take exams to become licensed and board certified as an attending physician in area of specialty.

Prepare for and take exams to become board certified and licensed as a general practitioner.

Specialty residency, or fellowship of three years in subspecialty such as gastroenterology or cardiology.

Prepare for and take exams to become licensed and board certified as an attending physician in area of subspecialty.

osteopathic manipulative treatment, which allows the body's healing systems to work freely. As you see from the chart, the levels of training are associated with different lengths of the white physician's coat. During medical school, students wear the shorter length white coat.

After Medical School

After the completion of medical school, new MDs or DOs have several options. The first and most common is to begin a three- to seven-year residency program in a field such as those listed on the chart. The American Board of Medical Specialties has a complete listing of all residency programs, also known as specialties, at www.abms.org. During this training, residents practice medicine under the supervision of fully licensed physicians, also known as attending physicians, in a private hospital or an academic medical center. They wear a mid-length white coat. First-year residents used to be known as interns, but now all residents are identified by postgraduate year: PGY-1, PGY-2, and PGY-3, and so on.

A second post–medical school option is the transitional year for MDs or DOs who have not been accepted into a residency program or who have to wait a year until a slot becomes available in the desired residency program. The transitional year program provides continuity of education and prepares the future resident for training.

The third post–medical school option is the one-year residency for general practitioners. One year of post–medical school training is required to apply for a permanent state license. Upon completion of training and licensing, new general practitioners can begin practicing without supervision as attending physicians, wearing the full-length white coats. General practitioners predated the family medicine residency program, which requires three years post–medical school training. General practitioners receive lower reimbursements and therefore command lower salaries.

After Residency

Upon completion of residency, physicians have two options. The first is to become licensed and board certified and begin practicing as attending physicians (in the full-length white coat). Board certification exams are much more grueling than the MCAT exam, taking two to three days. But they are also required throughout the physicians' training after years two and three in medical school and after the PGY-1 year. Physicians must meet state requirements, including a licensing exam, to become licensed. All physicians must be licensed to practice medicine. Physicians without board certifications can be licensed, but they cannot obtain hospital privileges.

Recertification and license renewal are required of all physicians periodically, varying by specialty and state. Internal-medicine practitioners must renew board certification every ten years, for example. Most states require continuing medical education (CME) as a condition for retaining licensure. Requirements vary by state. Alabama, for example, requires 25 hours per year of CME to include online programs, seminars, written information and audio and video resources.

The second post-residency option is to pursue a subspecialty by completing a fellowship of at least one year. Subspecialties such as cardiology, oncology, and gastroenterology follow an internal medicine residency. In rare instances, subspecialists such as oncologists can become even more specialized by developing expertise in treating one particular form of cancer. Fellows must become board certified and licensed if they have not already done so after completing their residency. Specialties with corresponding subspecialties are listed at www.abms.org.

The white coat length for a fellow depends on whether he is an attending in his specialty (for example, internal medicine) while training for a subspecialty (for example, nephrology) or he is receiving training and not practicing as an attending. A fellow who is not an attending wears a mid-length white coat. But some physicians choose to forgo the white coats altogether and wear scrub pants and tops for comfort and for less risk of spreading infection.

One field of medicine once considered alternative but now considered more mainstream is chiropractic care. DCs (doctors of chiropractic) have completed five years of postgraduate education in an accredited chiropractic program. DCs must complete at least a thousand hours of supervised clinical training and, like MDs, must become licensed and board certified and complete continuing education requirements. Chiropractors provide nonsurgical spinal care and can function as the quarterback in a team approach with physical therapists and orthopedic surgeons. Many states do not allow them to prescribe medicine or perform surgery, but they can coordinate care with MDs. They use techniques such as spinal manipulation, spinal adjustment, manual therapies for the joints and soft tissues, heat therapy, electrical modalities and rehabilitative exercises for pain management and maintenance.

Chiropractors are considered one type of primary health provider, meaning that they are a frontline provider. You do not need a referral to see a chiropractor, although MDs sometimes refer patients to DCs for conditions that respond better to chiropractic care.

Primary Care

The term *primary-care physician* usually conjures up visions of a general practitioner. What exactly is a primary-care physician? Again, a PCP is a frontline provider for whom you do not need a referral. The primary-care physician is the one who provides the referrals to specialists. In fact, many insurance plans require a referral from a PCP to a specialist. Your PCP is the quarterback for your entire medical team, including specialists, alternative practitioners, pharmacists, chiropractors, and physical therapists. Your PCP must act as the focal point, ensuring continuity of care and safety for you.

If you are seen at the emergency room, the ER personnel will ask, "Who is your primary-care physician?" Your PCP may admit you to the hospital and oversee your care, unless the hospital employs a hospitalist. A hospitalist functions as a PCP, but in a hospital setting. The hospitalist takes on the same role as your PCP while you are in the hospital. The purpose is to spare PCPs the long hours required to see patients in the clinic and in the hospital.

Your primary-care physician is probably an internist (doctor of internal medicine) or a family medicine practitioner, or possibly a general practitioner. Internists are better suited for older, less healthy patients, while family medicine specialists or general practitioners are a better fit for younger, healthier patients. Pediatricians are often PCPs for children, although family medicine specialists and internists can also treat children. Healthy women with few medical issues may see their obstetrician-gynecologists for primary care.

You may also opt to consult a nurse practitioner for primary care. Although nurse practitioners in 12 jurisdictions can practice independently, most work in a group practice. They are licensed by the state board of nursing and are registered nurses who have completed a master's degree in nursing and received advanced training in diagnosing and treating common medical conditions. Because their training includes an emphasis on nursing, their background allows them to look more at the art than the science of medicine. NPs often focus more on interpersonal skills and on treating the whole person. In many cases, they can spend more time with patients because they do not have to see as many patients in a day to make ends meet; they do not have the massive financial burden of medical school loans. NPs perform patient exams, order tests, diagnose conditions, prescribe medication, and in some cases, treat fractures and lacerations.

Physician assistants (PAs) provide many of the same services as nurse practitioners and are advanced clinicians who practice medicine with physician supervision. They have completed an accredited PA program lasting 24 to 36 months and 2000 hours of clinical rotations in family medicine, pediatrics, internal medicine, general surgery, emergency medicine, psychiatry, and obstetrics/gynecology. PAs are required to pass a certification exam administered by the National Commission on Certification of Physician Assistants (NCCPA) and to earn a hundred hours of continuing medical education every two years. They must be licensed by the state medical board. They conduct exams, diagnose and treat illnesses, assist with surgery, write prescriptions, and offer preventive counsel. Most physician assistants are found in a group physician practice or in a hospital setting. The single largest employer of PAs is the United States military (American Academy of Physician Assistants 2009).

NPs and PAs are becoming viable options for primary care as the internist and family practice shortages become more severe. Medical students are no longer attracted to these professions with lower incomes and long hours. The physicians who do practice internal or family medicine can only afford to accept a certain number of patients—usually 30 percent or less—with Medicare, Medicaid, or Tricare in order to make ends meet. These factors have created a primary-care crisis nationwide that will only get worse as the baby-boomer population ages.

As you can see, selecting a primary-care provider, or any medical practitioner, is a daunting task. First, you must find out if your practitioner of choice is taking patients and accepts your insurance plan. A quick way to narrow your options is calling the local or state medical society and asking which providers are taking new patients. To find medical societies in your state, visit www.ama-assn.org, click on Patients and the Medical Societies Directories tab. You will find a listing of all state medical societies, along with a listing of medical specialty societies, a vital resource in finding a specialist. Medical societies can also tell you if a practitioner is accepting Medicare, Medicaid, or Tricare.

Referrals and Insurance

You will probably need a referral from your PCP to a specialist. If your insurance provider does not require this, the specialist may. But this does not mean that you have to accept the choice dictated by your PCP and your insurance plan. There are ways around this, and there are more important factors than insurance coverage and PCP referrals, particularly for invasive procedures or life-threatening conditions. In her book *Fight Your Health Insurer and Win: Secrets of the Insurance Warrior*, Laurie Todd describes her fight for a referral to an out-of-network specialist and a more onerous battle for insurance coverage of the out-of-network treatment that ultimately saved her life. She literally fought for her life to obtain this treatment from the only specialist in the world who could adequately treat her rare form of cancer. Chapter 7 offers details on how Laurie accomplished this monumental task. As Laurie's experience shows, you have options.

Other Factors in Selecting a Practitioner

In addition to availability and insurance coverage, you need to consider many other factors when qualifying a medical practitioner. One of your best allies may be your pharmacist if you have a good relationship with her. Pharmacists hear the good, the bad, and the ugly when it comes to physicians, and they may share some of that information if they are comfortable doing so. If nothing else, your pharmacist can tell you which physicians have the best reputations and are easiest to work with. Nurses, lab and X-ray technicians, and pharmaceutical reps are also privy to physicians' reputations.

So what makes a good doctor? According to both the online Physician Survey and a survey conducted among lightning strike and electric shock patients, the overwhelming answer is listening skills. Medical practitioners often misunderstand or simply dismiss lightning and electric shock survivors because of the rarity of their injuries. These patients are especially passionate about finding a doctor who will listen and take them seriously.

You must be comfortable with your doctor, particularly your PCP. Doctors who enjoy people tend to practice in primary care or a specialty that allows for human interaction. The more reserved practitioners tend to gravitate toward a more analytical area such as surgery or radiology. In either case, you need a collaborative relationship, one that will allow you to participate equally in your care.

Your doctor should be accessible, especially your PCP. The best doctor in the world cannot help you if you cannot get an appointment for several weeks and if you cannot reach him in an emergency. The office staff is vitally important when considering a physician's accessibility. They are gatekeepers and control ease of access to your doctor. Accessibility is crucial in the event of an emergency. If your doctor is not available in the event of an emergency, law requires her to have coverage if she has admitting privileges and accepts private insurance. Because there are different levels of admitting privileges, you need to be clear on your doctor's privilege status.

Background checks are important, and you have several options for investigating doctors who behave badly. You can probe a physician's or a physician assistant's disciplinary history and verify licensure status by visiting the state medical board and doing a licensee search. You can find links to state medical boards at www.fsmb.org/directory_smb.html.

For a listing of state nursing boards, visit www.allnursingschools.com/
faqs/boards.php. For links to medical boards and other physician oversight organizations by state, visit www.consumerreports.org/health and
click on the Doctors and Hospitals tab, then select "Check up on your
doctor." At www.docfinder.org, you will also find links to state medical
boards, along with links to the AMA and the AOA (American Osteopathic Association).

Malpractice history is a double-edged sword. A physician, particularly a surgeon with a history of two or three prior claims against him,
may not be a safety threat. On the other hand, one physician managed
to practice in two different states with 120 malpractice claims against
him before this information became public and one of the state boards
recommended revoking his license. Now that is scary!

Online Information About Malpractice

The U.S. Department of Health and Human Services created the National Practitioner Data Bank (NPDB) to prevent inept or unprofessional
physicians and dentists from continuing to practice in multiple states.
The data bank includes history on physicians' and dentists' disciplinary
actions, malpractice judgments, and exclusion from participation in
Medicare and Medicaid.

There are a number of advantages to this safeguard, including a require-
ment for hospitals to query physicians before extending privileges to
them. You can learn more about the extent of protection by this data
bank at bhpr.hrsa.gov/dqa. Unfortunately, this data bank is not open
to the public and is only accessible to qualified entities, such as a hospital, a state medical board, or a professional society that performs
peer reviews.

HealthGrades recently launched an online physician malpractice database at www.healthgrades.com. Fifteen states provide malpractice
data: California, Connecticut, Florida, Idaho, Indiana, Massachusetts,
Maryland, North Dakota, New Jersey, New York, Oregon, Tennessee,

Virginia, Vermont, and West Virginia. HealthGrades provides basic physician information at no cost and charges $12.95 for a detailed report, including ratings and disciplinary actions during the last five years. Malpractice information is available for an additional $7.95. These costs are a very small investment considering the enormous risks posed by a proposed surgery.

Evaluating Credentials

Credentials are a key priority when selecting a medical practitioner. You can find a nurse practitioner at www.npfinder.com. Each state has varying licensure requirements for nurse practitioners, but all of them require national board certification. You can search online for your state nursing board and then do a licensee search within the site to verify that a nurse practitioner is licensed in that state. Physician assistant credentials are available at www.nccpa.net. Click on Verify PA-C to confirm the credentials of a nationally certified physician assistant. Most state medical board sites provide an option to do a licensee search for a physician assistant.

Chapter 4 lists several Web sites for searching physician credentials and patient ratings. For further investigation, visit www.abms.org to verify that a physician is board certified. You can even view a video on this site that describes the significance of board certification and how to select a physician. To find a physician's office with specialized credentialing, visit www.ncqa.org and click on "recognition" to see which physicians in your area have earned accreditation or certification for patient-centered medical home practices.

Checking Up on Surgeons

Surgeons' credentials deserve a special mention here. If someone is scheduled to cut into your body and perform delicate surgery, you need to make sure you have selected the best person for the job. Second and third opinions are absolutely appropriate in this situation. Not only is special caution needed in the event of a scheduled surgery, but surgery is sometimes avoidable.

Prior to any surgery involving joints or muscles, you may be wise to first exhaust all other options. Sometimes chiropractic care or physical therapy corrects the problem without surgery. Linda was advised to get arthroscopic surgery on her knee after severe pain forced her to wear a brace for weeks. She sought a second opinion and was referred to a physical therapist, who determined the origin of her pain in less than ten minutes. He explained that her longtime uneven gait, from arthritis pain in her hip, had caused one leg to compensate for the other, putting strain on the knee and causing the pain and swelling. Linda ultimately corrected the problem and found pain relief with physical therapy, completely avoiding surgery.

Surgeons perform amazing, lifesaving feats and deserve the utmost respect. But because of the risks associated with surgery, surgeons must be as experienced, qualified, and credentialed as possible. Surgeons are in their prime with five to twenty years of surgical experience. However, it's not just the years they put in, but also what they put into those years. If your surgeon of choice has five years of overall experience but been performing the surgery you need once a week for four years, she may be a better choice than a surgeon with eight years of overall experience but who performs the surgery you need only once a year.

If you need surgery for a rare condition, you might have to travel to find a surgeon specialized enough. You may require a sub-subspecialist, as Kristina from chapter 1 did. The only surgeon in Alabama with a surgical specialty for her condition performed her sphincter of Oddi surgery. He was a much better choice than a general surgeon who may only see this unusual condition once or twice in 30 years. But a general surgeon is a good choice for common surgery such as a cholecystectomy (gall bladder removal). Make sure you have the right surgeon for the right procedure. And, no, you should not completely defer this responsibility to your PCP, specialist, or surgeon. You can conduct online research, as Laurie Todd did to find the one specialist in the world who had a lifesaving protocol for her rare appendix cancer. If the only surgeon who can help you is not in your network, do you think you can count on help from your in-network providers?

The American College of Surgeons' (ACS) Web site, www.facs.org, covers this and many other topics thoroughly. Click on the Public and Press tab to find a plethora of vital information. Click on Information on Patient Choice, for complete information about your rights and choices as a patient. The Public and Press section provides information on surgeons' credentials with a recommendation to look for board certification and a fellowship in the American College of Surgeons, indicated by the initials FACS after a surgeon's name and MD title.

This section also offers tools for ensuring that the hospital where the surgeon has privileges is fully accredited. The Public and Press section lists common surgical procedures, recommendations for questions you should ask your surgeon, and a search tool for finding a surgeon with an ACS fellowship. From the Web site home page, you can also visit the Patients section for vital information on surgical specialties, preparation for surgery, and information about your organs and body systems.

Checking Up on Cancer Practitioners

Another area where selecting the right practitioner and treatment is absolutely critical is cancer. Because cancer and surgery are so intertwined, the ACS Web site covers cancer surgeries and treatments very thoroughly. Under Patient Resources, you can select Cancer to find detailed information on sixty different types of cancer, treatment guidelines for the most common cancers, a link to the clinical trials on the National Cancer Institute's Web site, and a partner site for the Commission on Cancer (CoC). The CoC accredits only the best cancer treatment facilities, just one in four hospitals. It has partnered with the American Cancer Society to create the National Cancer Data Base for the purpose of studying trends in cancer incidence and treatment. The data are available to the public at www.facs.org/cancer/ncdb/publicaccess.html.

Surgeons are part of the cancer treatment team, but the oncologist is the team's quarterback. An oncologist is the liaison, the central point of contact for a team that may include a surgeon or surgical oncologist, a radiation oncologist, a nutritionist, an alternative practitioner, and an interventional radiologist (one who implants a chemotherapy port and directs the chemo.) The makeup of the cancer team depends upon the type of cancer and the treatment needed. During my mother's battle with esophageal cancer, her team included her oncologist, a surgical oncologist (he put in her feeding tube and chemo port), a gastroenterologist who put a stent in her esophagus, a general surgeon to help with feeding tube issues, a nutritionist, and a natural pharmacist who recommended nutritional supplements.

Oncologists are most familiar with common cancers, such as breast, colon, and lung. But when the patient has a rare form of cancer, the oncologist will often recommend highly specialized treatment at a cancer specialty center or academic center. The type of center depends upon the type of cancer. The most well-known cancer centers are not always the best fit for certain rare cancers. Once again, some of the responsibility for learning about a lesser-known cancer, or any cancer for that matter, lies with the patient and the patient's support team. A cancer patient must have a support team to help with online research, everyday activities, emotional support, and getting to and from treatments.

The research is critical because there are so many different kinds of cancer that an oncologist who sees a rare cancer only once in her career may not be familiar with it. This is where peer-reviewed journals on Web sites such as PubMed, *New England Journal of Medicine*, and *Journal of the American Medical Association* are crucial sources of information for both patients and physicians. Additionally, patients and their support teams can find vital information on the sites listed in chapters 2 and 3, which include the American Cancer Society and the National Cancer Institute. The National Cancer Institute offers specific information on local resources at www.cancer.gov/cancertopics/factsheet/Support/resources and information on financial resources for cancer patients at www.cancer.gov/cancertopics/factsheet/Support/financial-resources. Oncologist Rachel Kruspe, MD, recommends Cancer Net (www.cancer.net), a site supported by the American Society of Clinical Oncology for comprehensive cancer information.

Considering Treatment Options

Choice of physician and treatment options is your right and your responsibility. Your options include the right to refuse treatment or to pursue an alternative treatment in favor of a mainstream treatment. Phyllis, a two-time cancer widow, has stated that she might decline chemotherapy if she were to develop cancer. She has every reason to feel that way after watching two husbands suffer through grueling cancer treatments of radiation and chemo, treatments that did not change the outcome.

Treatment, particularly chemotherapy, is a very individual decision. Many patients choose to fight cancer with medications that cause horrendous side effects. Those who are successful are glad they did. Even those who are not successful need to know they have done everything possible to beat the cancer. My mother never considered going down without a fight. She endured chemo until her oncologist gently told her that the cancer was spreading despite the treatments.

In retrospect, our family sees that he provided the optimal balance of cancer treatments and palliative care and allowed Mom to guide him in the direction that was best for her. He remained open to alternative supplements and to treatment at major cancer centers, although she was never strong enough to travel after her diagnosis. Mom fought her battle in a way that was best suited to her, the way that all patients should fight when battling life-threatening or life-limiting conditions.

The Experiences of Ivy and Karen

Ivy Larson was 22 years old when she developed what seemed like a chronic urinary tract infection, followed by embarrassing bouts of incontinence, irritating tingling and numbness in her leg, and ultimately urinary retention. The urinary retention episode landed her in the emergency room, and she soon received the devastating diagnosis of multiple sclerosis. MS is a disease that causes the immune system to attack the nervous system. The disease eroded the myelin sheath around Ivy's nerves, causing the numbness and urinary dysfunction.

Ivy had three choices for treatment: disease-modifying medication that alters the way the immune system works and that she would have to stop in the event of pregnancy; an experimental treatment; or the MS Diet, originally developed 60 years ago by Dr. Roy Swank. Ivy opted for the diet, the lowest risk option. Her symptoms began to disappear and she fully regained her life by following this low-fat healthy diet.

Her husband, Andrew Larson, MD, was fascinated by this phenomenon, and he and Ivy conducted their own research to create an updated nutrient-rich, anti-inflammatory whole food diet designed to prevent and reverse a number of diseases, such as heart disease, diabetes, asthma and allergies. This diet is the basis for their best-selling book *The Gold Coast Cure*. The Larsons continue to follow the anti-inflammatory diet and as a result, Ivy's multiple sclerosis has remained in remission for over a decade. Dr. Larson's blood pressure, body fat percentage, and energy levels have improved, and their eight-year-old son Blake has needed antibiotic treatment just once in his life.

Karen Grove became debilitated with fibromyalgia to the extent that she was almost completely bedridden. When traditional treatments did not work, she found the strength to seek her own treatment. She began to practice yoga and trained under Paul Jerard at Aura Yoga for one year and earned her hatha yoga certification. With his guidance, she learned to modify the moves in such a way as to help fibromyalgia sufferers without risking pain or injury.

As Karen continued to improve, she researched the effects of diet on fibromyalgia and found that certain foods, such as white flour and sugar, trigger pain attacks. She also found that what goes on the body is just as important as what goes into the body for fibromyalgia patients. She concluded that certain chemicals in cosmetics are irritants, and fibromyalgia patients must avoid them. Additional research led her to the pain-relieving effects of emu oil massaged into the skin and chiropractic adjustments specifically for fibromyalgia patients.

Based on her research, Karen made a number of lifestyle changes and improved so dramatically that today she is free of fibromyalgia symptoms. She developed a natural treatment regimen for fibromyalgia called the Grove Approach (www.thegroveapproach.com). Her protocol includes dietary guidelines, yoga instruction, chiropractic principles, psychological counseling, massage techniques, and her self-help book and cookbook.

Alternative treatments can be effective and natural. Both Ivy and Karen reclaimed their lives through safe, healthy, natural means. They did not have to try anything risky, and they did not take medication. Although I ultimately got my life back with allopathic treatment, as I mentioned earlier, I did enjoy a partial recovery for about 18 months from a very simple alternative treatment—power yoga.

One of My Treatment Choices

In 1998, when I was completely disabled with an undiagnosed condition and out of hope, I stumbled upon a magazine article about power-yoga instructor Mark Blanchard. Mark had suffered from a vestibular disorder caused by a ruptured eardrum, a result of a scuba-diving accident. His doctors told him that there were no treatments available to help him. On a hunch, he began practicing power yoga four hours a day, and his severe vertigo disappeared. A lightbulb flashed in my brain as I read the story. Although I knew I probably did not have a vestibular disorder, my symptoms were somewhat similar. I ordered Mark's first power-yoga video, *The Power Within*. Within four weeks, I saw very slight improvement and thought, *This can't be!* But I was not on any medication at that time and not attempting any other treatments. There was no other explanation.*

I continued to improve for another five months, reaching a functioning level of 50 percent. I was still unable to drive a car, but my brain tolerated stimuli better, and I could at least go into stores and restaurants with my driver. My memory lapses and lack of coordination were less noticeable. And that horrible, constant feeling of not being in my body was not as bad. I continued the workouts daily and enjoyed the higher functioning level for another year. Then all of a sudden, my body became accustomed to the workouts, and I regressed to my previous functioning level of about 25 percent. Although the power yoga was not a complete or permanent cure for my condition, it provided a much-improved quality of life for 18 months. That period of improved functioning gave me hope and helped me stay strong.

I recently contacted Mark Blanchard at his Los Angeles studio to find out if his power yoga workout (now expanded into a number of DVDs) has helped other medical conditions. He said, "Absolutely," citing the strong connection between mind and body. On a purely physiological

---

* As noted previously, for a Christian alternative to yoga, check out www.PraiseMoves.com.

level, yoga is very helpful for any condition that affects balance, such as vestibular disorders, proprioceptive disorders that affect the body's awareness in space. Yoga acts as a grounding agent for the body, helping the yoga practitioner feel rooted. Mark has also helped clients with cystic fibrosis, mild muscular dystrophy, and other muscular imbalances.

Help from Pilates

Pilates has healing properties because of benefits to the cardio-respiratory and lymphatic systems. Longtime Pilates instructor Dan Tripp helps his clients heal from a variety of illnesses and injuries, mostly neurological disorders and immune system dysfunctions. Dan is currently treating his own debilitating condition, Lyme disease, with regular exercise that includes Pilates, yoga, and qigong. He also practices meditation, receives gentle massage, and takes a number of supplements that contain fish oil. His objective is to keep his immune system as strong as possible to minimize the Lyme disease's flare-ups.

Dan credits Pilates as a potent preventive tool because of its core-strengthening effect and because it keeps the spine supple and less prone to degeneration and injury. Pilates, like yoga, is great for balance and flexibility, which are critical for mobility and preventing dangerous falls later in life. Both Pilates and yoga keep the body strong and balanced and also aid mind-body balance. Balance is important because, as Dan says, "An imbalanced body is at dis-ease."

The Alternative Medicine Option

What if you turn to an alternative protocol that is not as simple as diet or exercise? This is where it gets tricky. Alternative medicine is not nearly as regulated as traditional, or allopathic, medicine. We don't have as many credentialing organizations or other means to investigate alternative practitioners to make sure they practice safe medicine. Alternative practitioners typically do not have the 7 to 12 years of postgraduate training that allopathic practitioners have.

Does this mean alternative practitioners are less qualified and less able to help? Not necessarily. Alternative medicine certainly has a place in our health-care system, and the allopathic community tends to agree. In fact, the online Physician Survey revealed that 67 percent of the doctors surveyed are willing to coordinate care with an alternative practitioner if it is appropriate for the patient's situation.

Reputation is one of the best ways to find an alternative practitioner since those who treat patients successfully quickly develop a following. And some alternative practitioners are able to help when allopathic options have been exhausted, as Jordan Rubin's story in chapter 2 illustrates. Rubin was near death and his only possible option was a risky surgery. But Rubin sought a healthy, low-risk alternative regimen, and today he is a vibrant, healthy, successful author and natural health expert.

How can you possibly know which option is best—alternative or allopathic? One factor to consider is whether your condition is life threatening but has a fair to excellent prognosis with allopathic treatment. In this instance, allopathic treatment is the safer option, particularly in cases where time is of the essence, such as serious cardiac events. But in instances of chronic conditions like multiple sclerosis or fibromyalgia, and in the absence of a low-risk allopathic treatment, an alternative approach is worth consideration.

To pursue alternative treatment as safely as you can, arm yourself with as much information as possible and coordinate all alternative treatments with your PCP and any other physician whose treatment may be affected. The biggest danger lies in dangerous interactions between alternative and allopathic treatments. Chapter 3 lists online resources for investigating interactions between pharmaceutical medications, supplements and herbal remedies. Homeopathic remedies are very powerful and must be administered carefully by a trained homeopath and coordinated with all other medical treatments—alternative or allopathic.

When I became desperate to treat a stubborn, 18-month urinary tract infection, I showed Dr. Wyatt a number of unusual elixirs he had never seen, including an herbal blend I had ordered online that contained flying squirrel feces. He still hasn't let me live that down! The point is that desperation will prompt us to try anything and everything without proper precautions. That is why your PCP's participation is vital when you are investigating alternative options.

Fortunately, I found Ruth Kriz, a nurse practitioner who practices integrative medicine and specializes in chronic urinary tract infections after her own 11-year battle. Ruth and two microbiologists have researched chronic urinary tract infections extensively. They believe that what is known as interstitial cystitis is actually caused by a bartonella-like co-infection of Lyme disease and requires treatment with long-term antibiotics. Further, as an integrated practitioner, Ruth does not believe that antibiotics alone can treat the patient because the body must be in a state of optimal healing, so she orders tests for a number of vitamin and mineral deficiencies and treats those along with the infection. Eighty percent of her patients have improved significantly, and I am happy to be one of them.

An integrative practitioner like Ruth merges the best of both worlds. Alternative medicine is often a good complement to traditional medicine, which is why it is also known as complementary medicine. The National Center for Complementary and Alternative Medicine is part of the National Institutes of Health. You can learn more about it by visiting nccam.nih.gov. This site provides helpful tips on selecting a complementary practitioner and detailed information on herbal remedies and supplements.

An integrative practitioner or team of practitioners is an ideal choice if you are interested in pursuing alternative care. Another option is a formerly traditional practitioner who has transitioned into alternative care. Pharmacist Terry Wingo chose this path ten years ago; he closed his pharmacy and reopened it as a natural pharmacy. He made the choice because he was tired of seeing the same customers take the same medications for 20 years without getting better. He believed there had to be a better way, so he trained as a natural pharmacist and changed the course of his business and his life.

Terry sells a variety of supplements and herbal and homeopathic remedies, and he compounds both natural and pharmaceutical medications. He offers consultations to customers to make sure they are taking what they need, nothing more and nothing less. Both Terry and Ruth are passionate in their practice of functional medicine, the treatment of the underlying causes of illness rather than the symptoms. For more information, visit the Institute for Functional Medicine at www.functional medicine.org.

Alternative or allopathic, internal medicine or family medicine, surgeon or chiropractor—so many decisions. What should you do? Arm yourself with as much information as possible. Weigh the benefits and risks of all of your options. Assume your right and responsibility to find the best practitioner and the best treatment plan available. Release your inner proactive patient, and wield that power.

Chapter 6

When Good Hospitals Go Bad

Avoiding the Pitfalls and Taking Advantage of the Resources

David entered an esteemed teaching hospital to have his prostate surgically removed following a cancer diagnosis. As the surgical team prepared him for surgery, he noticed that they put marks on one of his legs. He mentioned it to his wife, and right before he was wheeled into the operating room, she checked his chart, where she saw the horrifying instructions—his leg was going to be amputated!

As it turned out, the charts for David and another patient with the same surname had been switched accidentally. The patient scheduled for the leg amputation was probably being prepped for prostate surgery. Fortunately, David's wife caught the error in time, and both men received the correct surgery. To make matters even worse, when David was recovering from his prostate surgery, his wife came into his hospital room and nearly sat on a full hypodermic needle that had been left in the chair.

Wrong-site and wrong-patient surgeries make headlines, but surgical errors occur even when patients have the correct surgery. Percy's (also a pseudonym) story is like something out of a bad television movie. The physician declared his original colonoscopy normal, despite the fact that Percy had been bleeding from the colon. Three months later, another colonoscopy revealed the presence of cancer 11 inches into the colon, and Percy underwent surgery to remove the cancer and resection his colon.

What should have been a routine, weeklong hospital stay turned into a month-long nightmare. During the surgery (a colectomy), Percy's ureter was cut accidentally, causing a dangerous condition known as hydronephrosis, an acute obstruction of the urinary tract that caused urine to back up into his kidney. This toxic condition caused Percy's system to shut down, and he suffered a heart attack the next day. He fought for his life for nearly 27 days in the hospital. Unfortunately, the physician and hospital staff never addressed the hydronephrosis.

Percy's family finally took him home, unaware of the hydronephrosis, only to rush him back to the hospital via ambulance ten days later when he hemorrhaged from his colon, losing six units of blood. The family requested a different team of physicians to address his serious complications. One discovered the hydronephrosis and placed a nephrostomy tube in his urinary tract to alleviate the complete obstruction. Another ordered two blood transfusions and a CT scan that revealed cancer metastases to the liver, the same cancer that the colonoscopy had not revealed several months earlier. Percy was advised to seek a possible liver resection at a larger teaching hospital, but he was too weak to undergo the surgery.

During the next several months, Percy had to be treated for urinary tract infections caused by the nephrostomy tube and had to have the tube changed. None of this suffering would have been necessary if not for the surgical error. And if the colon cancer had been caught during the first colonoscopy, his chances for beating the cancer might have been better. Instead, Percy suffered terribly during his last few months from the cancer and the hydronephrosis. He refused further hospitalization, opting instead for hospice care. He was unable to eat and needed morphine around the clock toward the end. He passed away 14 months after his surgery.

The same physician performed both colonoscopies and the surgery. Percy's son initiated a malpractice lawsuit against the physician and signed a fee agreement but did not hear anything from the law firm for the next four months. The day the statute of limitations expired, the son received a letter from the law firm stating that they could not take the case, citing lack of proof—despite the fact that Percy's hydronephrosis was clearly linked to the ureteral injury that occurred during his colectomy.

Adam (pseudonym) suffered a similar fate when he underwent surgery for advanced colon cancer. He anticipated the removal of his colon and a permanent colostomy, but he was not prepared for the horror he faced after surgery. The surgeon cut Adam's ureter during the surgery but tried to cover it up by calling in a urologist and claiming that the bladder had contained cancer. Rather than repairing the problem, he released Adam, who had a catheter and believed everything was okay. Once the catheter was removed, Adam quickly realized that he had no bladder control. He sought the help of a different urologist, who performed major surgery and discovered that the surgical error that had caused the ureteral injury had also cut off the blood supply to the bladder, urethra, and prostate.

As if that wasn't enough, Adam had developed a raging staphylococcus infection during his initial hospitalization. The urologist tried a number of procedures to save Adam's urinary organs, but ultimately he had to remove the bladder, urethra, and prostate. Adam had to wear a urostomy bag in addition to the colostomy bag, giving him very poor quality of life during his final two years. If the surgical team had corrected the error immediately, the organs probably would not have died and Adam could have retained normal urinary functioning during his last days. But instead, he suffered horribly, both physically and emotionally. Adam's widow, Chloe (pseudonym), filed a complaint with the state board of medical examiners, which found no basis for any action against the surgeon.

An Array of Errors

Hospitals are the scene of incredible lifesaving feats. Surgeons and their staffs deserve tremendous respect for the intricate work they perform. But physicians and hospital staff are human and prone to errors just like everyone else.

When we think of medical errors in hospitals, our thoughts turn immediately to surgical errors, which make headlines because they are either very serious, very bizarre, or both. Take, for example, the well-documented cases of three wrong-side brain surgeries at one hospital in less than a year or cases involving sponges or instruments left inside patients during surgery. A number of cases involve amputation of something the surgical team was not supposed to amputate.

Some errors that occur during surgery are related to anesthesia rather than the surgical process itself. Patients have reported terrifying instances of anesthetic awareness, or waking during surgery. This scenario is horrendous because the paralytic drugs work but the sedation fails. The patient hears and feels everything that is going on but is powerless to say or do anything. Talk about post-traumatic stress disorder! Anesthesia errors rarely result in death, with a rate of 1 in 13,000 reported in recent years (Lagasse 2002). However, that statistic is very significant for those who fall into the 1 rather than the 13,000. For more information on the anesthesia process, you can visit www.apsf.org or www.asahq.org/patientEducation.htm.

In addition to surgical errors, other adverse events occur in hospitals. These include drug-resistant infections caused by improper infection control; pressure sores; patient mix-ups; dietary mix-ups; falls; misdiagnosis; laboratory, X-ray, and pathology errors; and the number-one adverse event, medication errors. In the online Physician Survey, 50 percent of respondents named Medication Errors as the top hospital mistake; 32.6 percent selected Delays in the Emergency Department Waiting for Treatment; 4.3 percent chose Wrong-site Surgery; 4.3 percent picked Lab or X-ray Errors; and 8.7 percent cited Other Errors.

Harvard Medical School conducted a study in which researchers randomly chose 30,195 hospital records for review. Physician-reviewers studied the records of 1,133 patients who had suffered disabling injuries caused by medical treatment and found that medication errors, at 19 percent, were slightly more common than other adverse events (Leape et al., 1991). According to the Institute of Medicine, 1.5 million preventable adverse-drug events happen nationwide each year, with 50 percent taking place at transition points such as floor to operating room or hospital to nursing home.

Hospital medication errors include wrong medication, wrong dosage, medication delays, failure to notice drug allergies, and avoidable drug-to-drug interactions. Denise suffered a very serious but very preventable drug-to-drug interaction when she sought help at her hospital's emergency department. The physician and staff failed to notice which medications she was taking, and they administered a powerful pain reliever, with instructions to continue her regular medications. At home several hours later, Denise's mother checked on her and saw that she was incoherent and unable to stand up. Her mother called 9-1-1, and the paramedics had to resuscitate Denise during the two-mile ride to the hospital. Denise survived this egregious error only because her mother happened to check on her just in the nick of time.

Worrisome Statistics

Surgeon Atul Gawande, MD, MPH, offers unique insight into the fallibility of the medical profession and the perils of surgery in his book *Complications: A Surgeon's Notes on an Imperfect Science*. In 1999, the Institute of Medicine published a report entitled *To Err is Human: Building a Safer Health System*. According to this report, medical errors cause between 44,000 and 98,000 deaths per year in American hospitals, most of which are preventable. *The National Scorecard on U.S. Health Performance, 2008,* published by the Commonwealth Fund Commission on a High Performance Health System, reveals that the U.S. has the lowest ranking among 19 industrialized nations for preventing deaths with timely and effective care (Why 2008).

Addressing and Preventing Mistakes

Why do these errors occur? Fatigue, distractions, multitasking, patient handoff during shift changes and surgery, resident changes, miscommunication, and overworked physicians and staff all contribute to adverse events in hospitals. Dangerous errors are rarely attributable to just one person or process but instead are often the result of a combination of breakdowns in several individual processes that may have occurred over time, each without harm. But sometimes, the conditions are just right for a harmful event to occur.

The Institute for Healthcare Improvement (IHI) studies this phenomenon, using the Swiss cheese model designed by international human error authority James Reason. The premise of the Swiss cheese model is that a hazard must permeate multiple safeguards in order to cause harm. The Institute asserts that medical errors leading to patient harm actually consist of multiple errors. With each missed opportunity to catch an error, the chances increase that the error will slip through the barriers undetected and disaster will occur.

The Swiss cheese metaphor is helpful because if you line up several slices of Swiss cheese, the holes will probably not align, and you will not be able to pass a string through them. But if certain conditions are present, you can line up the holes. In a hospital, an adverse event can occur when a dangerous error slips through because a number of safeguards have holes in them.

For example, if a patient receives the wrong medication, there may be several errors involved. The problem may start with the physician's prescription for Celebrex for a patient in pain. The hospital pharmacy, feeling certain that the physician's handwriting says "Celexa," fills the prescription that way. After the nurse checks the patient's ID bracelet carefully, she tells the patient, "Here's your Celexa." The patient, who is a bit groggy, finds it odd that the doctor has prescribed a new drug but decides the doctor knows best and takes the medication. Several hours later, the patient, who regularly takes a monoamine oxidase inhibitor (MAOI), suffers a severe adverse reaction from the interaction between it and the Celexa, which cannot be taken safely with an MAOI. Throughout this process, nobody checked the list of the patient's current medications. So where did the system break down? Whose fault was it? This is an example of the Swiss cheese model, in which the holes line up perfectly to allow a multilevel system failure.

Learning from Experience and Observation

The Institute for Healthcare Improvement is committed to helping hospitals study errors and the environments that allow them. IHI advocates transparency and finding opportunities to learn from errors. The best-case scenario happens when the physicians and staff involved catch an error before it harms a patient, and then report it, so the entire hospital team can learn from the error. But in some cases, a patient is harmed, and physicians and staff may be less than forthcoming for fear of consequences. IHI recommends creating an environment of mutual trust in which physicians and staff can report harmful errors without fear of reprisal.

This may sound counterintuitive—after all, a health-care professional who harms a patient should be punished, right? Unfortunately, if a health-care professional fears serious consequences, he is much less likely to speak up. If medical errors are not identified, they cannot be corrected, and future patients are vulnerable. IHI takes the position that it is in everyone's best interest to create an environment in which errors are transparent. That's not to say that health-care professionals with a pattern of errors should not be subject to punitive action. But researchers must study unintentional human errors not tied to a performance problem as part of ongoing patient safety initiatives.

IHI provides a number of avenues available to hospitals and physicians' offices for creating a culture of safety. They encouraged health-care professionals worldwide to participate in their 5 Million Lives Campaign, which challenged health-care professionals to save five million patients from harm from December 2006 to December 2008 and resulted in 122,000 fewer fatalities during that period. IHI presents several seminars throughout the year, along with an annual conference. The Web site, www.ihi.org, offers mini-courses online on patient safety through IHI Open School, as well as information on a number of timely health-care topics. IHI also provides fellowship training for select health-care practitioners interested in more intensive training.

Accrediting and Overseeing Hospitals

Another organization heavily invested in patient safety is the Joint Commission (www.jointcommission.org), an oversight organization that is the gold standard in hospital accreditation. In order for a hospital to receive and maintain Joint Commission accreditation, it must undergo a rigorous process called a survey every 18 to 39 months. The survey can last two or three days for smaller hospitals and five days for larger hospitals. The number of surveyors depends on hospital size, extending to five for large hospitals. In the past, the Joint Commission informed hospitals ahead of time of a survey, now surveys are unannounced.

During the survey, the Commission looks for compliance with a comprehensive set of standards related to patient safety and quality of care. If the hospital has a successful survey, it is then accredited for a three-year period. The Joint Commission's accreditation also offers hospitals "deemed status." Deemed status indicates that the organization is in compliance with the Centers for Medicare and Medicaid Services' (CMS) conditions of participation. Deemed status is required in order for a hospital to be reimbursed for services provided to Medicare patients.

The Joint Commission is one accreditation organization (AO) that offers accreditation and deemed status. Others include DNV and the American Osteopathic Association. The Joint Commission also offers accreditation to ambulatory-care facilities, behavioral health-care facilities, home health-care organizations, laboratory services, long-term care facilities, and office-based surgery centers. Hospitals and other facilities that do not use an accreditation organization (AO) are surveyed by their state department of public health. These surveys are conducted less frequently than surveys by an AO. In most states facilities surveyed by an AO are exempt from accreditation surveys by the state department of health.

Aside from the obvious CMS reimbursement issue, why do hospitals subject themselves to the anguish of the accreditation process, particularly the more frequent surveys by AOs? It is the right thing to do for the patients, and it makes good business sense. Looking at the bottom line, hospitals cannot afford to allow hazards to remain undetected, given the threat of malpractice litigation, bad publicity, and stiff fines for health code violations from state departments of health services.

CMS recently imposed a harsh penalty by refusing to cover serious preventable events and including a stipulation that hospitals cannot bill patients for them. Preventable events fall into three categories: wrong surgical or other invasive procedures performed on a patient, surgical or other invasive procedures performed on the wrong body part, and surgical or other invasive procedures performed on the wrong patient (CMS 2009). CMS can also request a validation survey of a hospital or other facility, to ensure the thoroughness of an AO accreditation survey. The validation survey is conducted by the state health department.

How Hospitals Improve

Hospitals must exercise a strong commitment to quality care and safety for patients. The Joint Commission is there not just to investigate, but also to guide physicians and hospitals, offering numerous tools for creating a safe and efficient environment. One of these tools is the National Patient Safety Goals (www.jointcommission.org/PatientSafety/ NationalPatientSafetyGoals). Another is the Universal Protocol at www .jointcommission.org/PatientSafety/UniversalProtocol. The Joint Commission's Universal Protocol aids organizations in the prevention of wrong-site, wrong-procedure or wrong-person surgery.

The World Health Organization recommends a surgical safety checklist to reduce the risk of surgical errors. To learn more about this checklist in action, you can visit www.safesurg.org and scroll to the videos at the bottom of the page. The videos present examples of a surgical checklist administered both correctly and incorrectly. This site also provides the World Health Organization's surgical safety checklist. The WHO conducted a study to determine the impact of its checklist and found that this vital tool reduced the rate of deaths and complications by more than one third (Gawande et al., 2009, 491-499). Each individual hospital can and should tailor the checklists provided by the World Health Organization and the Joint Commission to meet its own needs and culture.

Reputable hospitals and surgical centers use safeguards such as the Universal Protocol or the WHO Checklist and employ other preventive measures such as patient ID bracelets and color-coded wristbands to identify patients' drug allergies and patients at risk of falling. The color codes vary from one hospital to another, but many Alabama hospitals use red bracelets to identify patients with drug allergies, yellow for fall risks, and purple for "do not resuscitate" orders. The color-coded wristbands are especially helpful given the number of patient handoffs and transports that take place in hospitals.

Medication reconciliation substantially reduces medication errors when using a multidisciplinary approach based on an electronic system (Agrawal and Wu 2009). The Joint Commission requires organizations to have a procedure in place for medication reconciliation, the process of comparing a patient's current medications with those ordered for the patient while under the care of the hospital. Medication reconciliation is performed when a patient is admitted to the hospital and any time the patient is transferred within the hospital to a different level of care, for example from the intensive care unit (ICU) to a non-ICU room, or to another health-care organization such as a long-term-care facility. When a patient is discharged, she is provided a complete list of her medications and it is explained to her. This list also is given to the patient's doctor who will primarily be responsible for her care.

Computerized physician order entry (CPOE) is one tool for medication reconciliation. CPOE takes the mystery out of the physician's handwriting because it enters all physicians' orders, including medication, into a computer system and makes them available to all staff hospital-wide. Bar code medication administration (BCMA) technology is also helpful for safer medication administration. BCMA helps to ensure that the right medication gets administered to the right patient, usually by scanning a bar code on the patient's ID wristband. Although technology offers protection against medication errors, systems are only as good as the people who use them. Hospitals must commit not only to the purchase of expensive electronic systems, but also to training for all members of the hospital staff and to periodic audits to ensure that staff members are using the systems properly.

Nurses play an important role in safe medication administration. In nursing school, they receive training on the five rights of patients: right patient, right route, right dose, right time, right medication. Nurses are often the liaison between the patient, physician, and pharmacy, making them a vital role in the process, and they have other critical responsibilities, including resuscitating patients. Nurses are more likely than physicians to be close by when a patient stops breathing. They must think and act very quickly while getting hit with pressure from all sides—patients, physicians, pharmacy, lab personnel, and hospital administration, in some cases.

Members of the Health-Care Team

Who are all the people who come into your hospital room at all hours, and what do the initials behind their names mean? An RN is a registered nurse who has completed two to four years of education. An LPN or LVN is a licensed practical nurse or licensed vocational nurse and has typically completed one to two years of education.

A nurse's assistant or nurse technician has completed a certificate program. They all work closely with one another and the rest of the health-care team.

Other members of your health-care team may include an X-ray technician, who has completed three to four years of education, and a phlebotomist (draws blood), who has completed six months of training. If you encounter any problems with your hospital care or continuity care, you can ask for the charge nurse, who functions as a manager on duty for the nursing team.

The Patient Advocate

A significant hospital role is that of the patient advocate. Many hospitals employ at least one. I asked Robbin McCord, quality coordinator and safety officer at Huntsville Hospital in Alabama, how many patient advocates his hospital employs. He responded, "We're all patient advocates," and proceeded to describe the duties of the hospital's full-time advocate. Ideally, all hospitals would share this philosophy while at the same time engaging at least one full-time patient advocate, patient liaison representative, or patient ombudsman. Patient advocates are vital not only to patient safety, but also to quality of care.

While my mother was a patient at West Virginia University Hospital a month before she passed away, Dad and I found the patient advocate service very helpful. Mom needed medication to help make her more comfortable, but it could not be administered safely until a clostridium difficile bacterial infection had been ruled out. The lab's busy schedule meant it could not process the test for two days. Dad and I consulted the patient advocate, and two hours later, the test had been expedited and Mom had her medication. This may sound like a small step, but it made a huge difference in Mom's comfort during her final weeks. We were so grateful that the hospital employed someone who knew the inner workings of the hospital and could expedite the process.

A patient advocate does not have a magic wand or, in many cases, a medical background. According to Erin Waddell, patient advocate at Fairmont General Hospital in West Virginia, a patient advocate is a liaison between the patient and the hospital's health-care providers. She must stay neutral and exercise a great deal of diplomacy in all dealings. She must maintain good working relationships with directors and managers in order to call on their departments when a patient needs help. She handles problems ranging from long wait times in the ER to physician behavior to accounting questions. In most cases, patients want to vent, and they want someone to listen, even if the advocate cannot help. But often she can help because her relationship with the various departments allows her to get problems resolved quickly. If a hospital is especially transparent, the administration will ask for ongoing reports from the advocate to identify problems within the hospital.

You can benefit from the services of a patient advocate in any area of the hospital: inpatient, outpatient, and emergency department. In the ER, you can use the house phone to call the patient advocate. If the hospital does not employ an advocate, you can ask for the hospital administrator. As an outpatient, you can use the house phone or ask a staff member. The same procedure applies if you are an inpatient. The patient advocate will call or visit your hospital room unless you have a friend or family member who can go to the advocate's office.

If a hospital employs a patient advocate, it will list contact information in the packet of information you receive upon admission. The hospital should also display this information on its Web site. The hospital switchboard operator can connect you to the patient advocate's phone.

In addition to seeking help from the charge nurse, hospital administrator, or patient advocate, there are a number of other actions you can take to help ensure a safe and comfortable hospital stay. Visit www.joint commission.org/PatientSafety/SpeakUp for brochures on prevention of infection, medical testing mistakes, avoidance of surgery mistakes, and follow-up care after discharge. You can find a number of valuable patient fact sheets on hospitalization and general health topics at www.partner shipforhealthcare.org/resources/factsheets.asp.

Managing Your Hospital Stay

Chapter 5 provides tips for qualifying your surgeon. But equally important is qualifying the hospital where you will undergo surgery or receive treatment by using the following measures:

- If your physician has privileges at more than one hospital, ask which hospital she recommends and why. She will have insight into the safety culture of each hospital.

- Weigh benefits and risks of hospitals versus surgery centers for outpatient surgery. Hospitals are safer for any procedure done under anesthesia and for any procedure that could cause dangerous complications. If something goes wrong with the surgery or anesthesia, you need a facility equipped to handle the emergency.

- If you have options, select a larger hospital that offers a variety of treatments and surgeries, or a teaching hospital. If you are scheduled for surgery, make sure the hospital performs this procedure on a regular basis. Your surgeon or the hospital quality assurance manager can provide information about its experience with your type of surgery.

- Check hospital credentials, licensing, ratings, and infection rates. Hospitals make accreditation information available on their Web sites, in their patient literature, posted in their hallways, or any combination of the above. To find a Joint Commission–accredited organization, visit www.QualityCheck.org. You can check with your state department of health services to ensure that the hospital is licensed, and you can visit www.leapfrog group.org/for_consumers, www.healthgrades.com, or www .hospitalcompare.hhs.gov for hospital ratings. The hospital's quality assurance manager has statistics on infection rates.

- Stay current with media coverage of local hospitals. The media typically expose errors such as a wrong-site surgery or a methicillin-resistant staphylococcus aureus (MRSA) outbreak. MRSA is a strain of staph that is resistant to most antibiotics, and in some cases it is fatal. Most hospitals do not volunteer this information freely.

- If possible, select a hospital with sophisticated equipment, including electronic records. Again, your surgeon or PCP will have this information, as will the hospital's quality assurance manager.

- Avoid a hospital stay during the weekend and the summer months, if possible. Weekend admissions are associated with higher mortality rates than weekday admissions because of lower staffing levels (Bell and Redelmeier 2001). In teaching hospitals, mortality rates are higher from July through September, when new medical school graduates start residency training. Shift changes are another dangerous time in hospitals because of patient handoffs.

Prior to hospitalization, you need to clarify who will be in charge of your care. If you are scheduled for surgery, your surgeon will be the attending physician, or the physician in charge. If your hospital stay is not surgery-related, in most cases your PCP or a hospitalist will be the attending physician. Your attending physician may call in a specialist, who will be the consulting physician. At any rate, you need to know who is in charge.

Be sure your attending physician and your advocate (a friend or family member) have your medical history, including medications and drug allergies. Remember the lists in chapters 3 and 4? They will come in mighty handy during your hospitalization. You should pack your lists in your overnight bag, along with your needed medications. (Some hospitals do not allow patients to keep medication in their rooms, but what if the hospital does not have a needed medication in stock? If you are not sedated, your attending physician may sign an order allowing you to administer your own medication.)

Getting Ready to Undergo Surgery

If you are scheduled for surgery, the time to ask the bulk of your questions is during the office visit prior to the surgery. You will need to ask your surgeon the following:

- Are there any alternatives to surgery?
- What are my presurgery instructions?
- How long will I have to stay in the hospital?
- What will be done to prevent postsurgical infection (for example, antibiotics) and blood clots (for example, compression hose)?
- Are procedures in place in the event of dangerous complications?
- What kind of surgical checklist is used?
- What will I need to do after surgery to gain the most benefit from the surgery?
- What are my limitations after surgery?
- How long is the expected recovery time?

For additional information on preparation for surgery, Thomas Russell, MD, executive director of the American College of Surgeons, offers valuable insight, tools, and tips in his book *I Need an Operation…Now What? A Patient's Guide to a Safe and Successful Outcome.*

Once you are in the hospital, your advocate will need to stay with you if you are going to be sedated. If you are undergoing surgery, your advocate will need to speak to the surgeon while you are in recovery, and she will need to be with you when you wake up or when you are admitted to a hospital room. She should carry a notebook to jot down comments from the surgeon and other doctors and nurses who come in to see you.

Just before surgery, you will have a chance to ask the surgeon and the anesthesiologist any questions you might have. This is a good time to request that the surgeon mark the surgery himself in the pre-procedure area. Be sure to verify three very important identifiers with the surgical staff: right person, right surgery, and right body part. Tell the anesthesiologist if you have had any difficulty with anesthesia before, such as nausea. And remember, minor surgery is when it is happening to someone else; major surgery is when it is happening to you.

Maintaining Vigilance

Once you settle into your hospital room, you and your advocate must be vigilant. Do not take any medication administered by anyone who fails to check your ID bracelet first. Don't be afraid to speak up and ask for the name and purpose of the medication. Do not allow any hospital staff member to touch you without first donning gloves or washing her hands. Hospital-acquired infections, particularly MRSA, are on the rise. Because health-care workers are exposed to so much illness, your risk is elevated by close contact with them, especially in a hospital setting.

Be mindful of your right to know the role of everyone who provides care while you are in the hospital. When it comes to your body, you have the right to know who is doing what and why. If you are concerned about any aspect of your care, don't hesitate to call the patient advocate or administrator. If you are not satisfied after following proper protocol within the hospital system, you can contact the accreditation organization or state department of public health.

Prior to discharge from the hospital, make sure you understand clearly all of your after-care instructions. During your final consultation in the hospital with your physician, ask specific questions about activities that you can resume or must avoid. Clarify dietary requirements and limitations. If you have had surgery, make sure you understand proper care of the surgical site and other steps you can take to prevent infection. If you require extended treatment such as physical therapy or a stay in a rehabilitation hospital, ask to speak with a case manager or a social worker who can help you navigate the process.

When You Have to Visit the ER

The above suggestions are helpful for a planned hospitalization, but what about an admission through the emergency department? Or any visit to the emergency department for that matter? ER visits are rarely planned, which is yet another reason advance preparation is needed. In addition to keeping medication and medical history up to date and handy, your most powerful tool for getting the best emergency care is knowing your options before you have a medical emergency. The worst time to explore your options is in the midst of a possible cardiac event, while bleeding profusely, or while vomiting uncontrollably.

ER visits can range from uncomfortable to miserable to downright dangerous. Two years ago, I had to visit the ER while traveling out of state. Despite the fact that I had chest pain and difficulty staying conscious, the triage nurse decided, based on my vitals, that I was not "fast track." For the next six and a half hours, I struggled to stay conscious while sitting in the waiting room. The ER staff could not provide a place for me to lie down, and when I had to lie on the floor because I was having difficulty staying conscious, a nurse told me that was against hospital policy. She offered a wheelchair and performed an EKG in a room off the waiting room to rule out a heart attack.

After three hours, I called an urgent care clinic and was told that if I had presented with those symptoms at their facility, I would have been given IV fluids and transported to the same hospital by ambulance. I considered leaving the ER and doing just that, but I was concerned that my insurance provider would not cover the EKG if I left before treatment was completed. So I continued to wait while watching fast-track patients who arrived long after I did walking without difficulty back to the exam rooms when the nurse called their names. When I finally saw the ER physician after the long wait, he determined that I was suffering from dehydration, as I had suspected, and admitted me for 24-hour observation and IV fluids.

As a result of this experience, I avoid emergency departments whenever I have a dehydration episode. If I am able to drive safely and sit in a chair, I go to a nearby urgent care facility, where I usually wait thirty minutes or less in the waiting room. As soon as the nurse calls me back to the exam room and gets my vitals, she starts the IV fluids. I receive two or three bags of fluid and meet with the physician while getting them. The urgent care staff tries to put the IV in my hand so I can bend my arm, checks on me periodically, and brings me warm blankets. They don't mind if I bring my laptop; in fact, I wrote portions of this book in their facility.

When I am not able to drive and not able to sit in an ER waiting room, I request a direct hospital admission. That way, I get the care I need without the time in the ER waiting room. As soon as I have a confirmed admission, I pack an overnight bag and call a friend to drive me to the hospital one mile from my home. We get a wheelchair at the door (my blood pressure is usually around 70/40 in these instances), and I am wheeled to admissions and then to a room, where I receive IV fluids and get blood work and an EKG. Fortunately, the dehydration episodes have abated since Dr. Watkins, my autonomic disorders specialist, increased my Zoloft and Florinef dosages to help my body use fluids more efficiently.

If you have a chronic condition that requires periodic hospitalization, I highly recommend this approach. If the hospital admissions office has not closed for the day, any physician with hospital privileges can do a direct admission. If you and your physician know that you will need hospitalization, it makes sense to bypass the emergency department, where you will be more exposed to illness. According to Robert Lesslie, MD, a 25-year veteran emergency department physician, the ER waiting room is the most dangerous area of the hospital.

If you are admitted to the hospital, your PCP, a hospitalist, or the emergency department physician will probably admit you. In some cases, a specialist or subspecialist may do it. Unfortunately, fewer PCPs are admitting patients and seeing them in the hospital. If your PCP does not see patients in the hospital, your attending physician will probably be a hospitalist. You may receive care from a resident under supervision from an attending physician if you are admitted to a teaching hospital.

The ER vs. Urgent Care

When weighing the pros and cons of the ER versus an urgent care clinic, consider the severity of your condition and whether or not an urgent care clinic has the resources to treat your condition. At the very least, call the facility to find out which diagnostic and treatment options are available before you. Better yet, contact urgent care clinics when you are not having an emergency to find out which emergency services they cover and which insurance plans they accept. If your emergency is late at night and you cannot wait until the next morning, the ER is your only choice unless you have access to a 24-hour urgent care clinic. Critical emergencies that must be addressed in emergency department include...

- chest pain
- shortness of breath
- heavy bleeding
- severe, unusual headache
- high fever
- loss of consciousness
- stroke symptoms such as numbness, confusion, or slurred speech
- inability to walk or stand due to symptoms
- any sudden, unusual debilitating symptom
- major broken bones
- stabbings and gunshot wounds

Most of these symptoms warrant a call to 9-1-1 for an ambulance. Don't wait until you have an emergency to find out whether your insurance covers ambulance transportation. In an emergency, you do not have time to worry about such matters. If you are having a true emergency, arrival in an ambulance will get you to an exam room much more quickly. More important, the paramedics can radio ahead to the ER staff to give them your vitals and let them know what to expect. The paramedics can also start treatment right away, which often means the difference between life and death.

If you are not having a true emergency and call an ambulance in an effort to shorten the wait time, the ER staff will probably catch on and escort you to the waiting room. Ditto for faking a seizure or a fainting spell. My sources tell me that ER personnel are trained to detect faking. Vomiting and bleeding in some ERs will command attention more quickly, for the greater good if nothing else. Other patients do not want to see it, and it just plain looks bad for the hospital.

Less critical emergencies that are more appropriate for urgent-care clinics include...

- broken bones
- cuts requiring stitches

- IV fluids

- bad flu or respiratory infection

- asthma attacks or allergic reactions that don't threaten breathing

What to Expect in the ER

Clearly, an emergency department visit is a last resort, but sometimes necessary. Why are some ERs better than others? It depends on the hospital's culture and the hospital administration's mind-set. If the top administrators recognize the fiscal value of the emergency department, which is responsible for 15 to 20 percent of most hospital admissions, they are more likely to allocate resources to it. Unfortunately, many hospital administrators view the emergency department as a sinkhole and treat it as such, an attitude that leads to understaffed and overcrowded ERs.

Adding to the chaos of the ER is the fact that many patients use it for primary care. Some do so because they do not have medical insurance and thus have limited options. Others do so because they cannot find a PCP given the shortages of internists, family medicine doctors, and pediatricians. This is why urgent care clinics are a viable option for those with medical insurance coverage and emergencies that are not life threatening.

If you must seek treatment in an emergency department, what can you expect? If you don't arrive by ambulance, you can expect a triage nurse to call you once you have signed in. After you present your insurance card (first things first), they will assess you to determine your level of acuity (the severity of your symptoms). Most ERs use a scale ranging from 1 to 5 to determine level of acuity. For example:

1. Most serious, intervention needed ASAP (for example, cardiac cases)

2. Requires intervention within 30 minutes (for example, most car accidents, severe asthma)

3. Requires two or more resources (for example, infant with fever)

4. Sutures or X-rays required (for example, injuries in which bleeding has stopped)

5. Least severe, needs oral medication (for example, flu without heavy vomiting)

Many emergency departments have a protocol for assessing patients in a private treatment area (PTA) adjacent to the waiting room after taking vitals. In this area, the patient receives tests such as EKG, X-rays, blood work, or a strep tests. Some PTAs are even equipped for starting IV fluids. The more services the PTA provides, the more quickly patient traffic flows in the emergency department.

To make your visit to the hospital emergency department as safe and efficient as possible, consider doing the following.

Ways to Help the ER Help You

Contact your PCP before heading to the ER. If she is a staff physician and knows your history, she may be able to do a direct admission and bypass the emergency department. Although it is highly unlikely, she may meet you at the ER. Instead, she will probably call the ER to let them know you are on your way. She can contact the PTA and order lab work and other tests to expedite the diagnostic process. If you are in acute distress, call 9-1-1 first and then your PCP.

Gather as much history as possible to take with you. The ER staff can help you much more efficiently if you have your lists of medications and drug allergies, past hospitalizations and surgeries, chronic conditions, and immunizations (particularly for children) with you, along with legal paperwork such as a living will and advanced directive. In a sudden, life-threatening emergency, you will not be able to gather all of this information. This is where the wallet card mentioned in chapter 3 comes in handy. You might also consider carrying a flash drive with your medical records on it when you are traveling.

Ask for help with your symptoms during your wait. If you are vomiting, ask for an injection of antinausea medication. If your pain is unbearable, ask for pain medication. If you need desperately to lie down and there are no beds available, ask the triage nurse if there is a consultation room with a sofa. Many emergency departments have a consultation room for meetings between ER staff and patients' families.

Expect a longer wait during peak times. Emergency departments are busiest during the evenings and early mornings, and also on weekends and holidays. Winter months are busier because of flu season.

Be assertive, but be respectful. ER physicians, nurses, and administrative staff have chosen extremely stressful professions. They encounter blood and guts regularly. They often have to tell family members their loved ones didn't make it. And perhaps their most heart-wrenching responsibility is assessing and treating defenseless child abuse victims. Many ER physicians burn out after ten years. (Dr. Robert Lesslie offers keen insight into the chaotic lives of ER physicians and staff in his book *Angels in the ER.*) You will not get very far if you vent your frustrations on the ER staff. If the system is not working, the fault probably lies within the hospital administration. If you are not happy with your treatment in the ER, use the house phone to call the patient advocate or administrator on duty.

Understand your risks if you leave without full treatment. If you get tired of waiting for hours in the emergency department and choose to leave, you will be asked to sign a waiver. Before you sign the waiver, ask if the hospital will bill you. If it does, your insurance provider may not cover the cost of whatever services you received (vitals in triage, EKG), and you will be stuck with the bill. If you receive this type of bill, call the hospital's patient advocate and explain your situation. Most hospitals would rather waive that kind of bill than risk bad publicity.

Know which hospitals your insurance plan covers. You need to know before you have an emergency. If you seek treatment at an out-of-network hospital, you may be penalized, particularly if an in-network hospital is nearby. Study your plan to determine your options in the event of a medical emergency while traveling. You will not have time to worry about these matters when an emergency occurs.

Hospitals have their risks, but the good far outweighs the bad. In a perfect world, we could expect flawless surgeries, infection-free hospitalization, medication administered free of errors, and short waiting times in the emergency department. In the real world, adverse events are possible but less likely when patients, physicians, hospitals, and oversight organizations are all working together.

Chapter 7

"Someone Took Away
Our Swords," Part One

Finding Success with Insurance Providers

The women sat in a circle during a support group meeting at the annual Lightning Strike and Electric Shock Survivors International conference. One by one, they told wrenching tales of medical insurance battles, or worse, no medical insurance at all. They described roadblocks in obtaining disability compensation and workers' compensation despite obvious disabling symptoms. They discussed the challenges of facing not only their physical symptoms, but all of the secondary difficulties that accompany them. Their injuries left them unable to work and unable to qualify for disability or workers' compensation because of a constellation of symptoms that nobody understands.

Most physicians do not see even one lightning or electric shock injury during their entire career and, therefore, do not have the incentive to understand such an injury. Only a handful of physicians across the country knows how to treat these injuries, making it very difficult for survivors to receive proper treatment. To make matter worse, many physicians refuse to acknowledge this kind of injury, which causes a multitude of problems. Without the all-important physician verification of a disabling condition, patients have a very slim chance to qualify for disability or workers' compensation. Without compensation, there is no income, no medical insurance, and no hope of getting better. Lightning and electric shock survivors are especially vulnerable to this calamity of no compensation and often feel as though they are fighting a fierce battle completely unarmed. During the support group meeting, Marianne, a lightning survivor, spoke up and said, "It feels like someone took away our swords."

If you are suffering from a catastrophic illness or injury, you know exactly how it feels to fight this battle unarmed. It's bad enough that you have to cope with debilitating or painful symptoms or both. But when you have to battle your insurance provider constantly, if you are fortunate enough to have an insurer, you may feel as though insult has been added to injury. If you are suffering through the rigorous application for disability or workers' compensation, you have probably been labeled unfairly as a malingerer. You have undoubtedly appealed an unfavorable decision at least once and completed mounds of paperwork. The battles associated with medical insurance, disability, and workers' compensation providers are difficult enough for healthy people. How are people battling illness or injury expected to cope with these challenges?

Providers Who Don't Want to Provide

Medical insurance coverage in the United States leaves much to be desired. In the movie *Sicko*, director Michael Moore's opening interviews are with unfortunate patients forced to forgo necessary medical treatment because they have no health insurance. The movie underscores the fact that nearly 50 million Americans are not covered by medical insurance and 18,000 per year die because they lack medical care. The Commonwealth Fund Commission on a High Performance Health System concurs in its "National Scorecard on U.S. Health System Performance, 2008." Its study reports that 42 percent of all working-age adults are uninsured or underinsured and gives the U.S. a score of 58 out of 100 for insurance and access (Why 2008). The World Health Organization reports that despite poor health-care coverage nationwide, the U.S. spent 15.3 percent of its gross domestic product on health care in 2006 (United States 2009).

In *Sicko*, after illustrating the plight of the uninsured, Moore announces that the movie is not about people without insurance—it is about those who have it. Frighteningly, they don't fare much better. One couple who appears in *Sicko* became homeless after the husband had a heart attack and the wife developed cancer. Their co-pays and deductibles reached such astronomical heights that they were forced to sell their home, declare bankruptcy, and move in with their daughter.

Moore interviews several patients who were denied coverage by their insurance providers ostensibly because treatments were "experimental," "out of network," "not preapproved," or "not medically necessary" or because of a pre-existing condition clause. A woman who was hit by a car traveling at 45 miles per hour had to pay for ambulance service out of pocket. Her insurer rejected her claim because the ambulance ride was not preapproved. She could not call for preapproval because she was unconscious when paramedics transported her to the hospital.

A man describes his frustration while seeking cochlear implants for his hearing-impaired infant daughter. The insurance company initially agreed to pay for just one ear, claiming that the procedure for the second ear was experimental. When he threatened the insurance provider with adverse publicity, the provider relented and covered the implants for both ears. A young woman could not get coverage for cervical cancer treatment after her insurance provider issued the edict that she was too young to have cancer. She ended up cancer-free but badly in debt and sought subsequent medical care in Canada.

Other cases Moore presents end much more tragically. A man with kidney cancer died without treatment because his insurer repeatedly denied coverage for every kind of treatment that would have helped him and deemed a lifesaving bone-marrow transplant experimental. A large HMO refused to cover testing and treatment for an infant rushed to the nearest hospital with a 104-degree temperature. Because the hospital was not in the insurer's network, the emergency department sent the infant and her mother to an in-network hospital. The little girl died because of the delay in treatment.

Taking the Hit

In *Sicko*, Moore also interviews former insurance-company executives who had been tasked with finding any loophole, no matter how harsh, to avoid paying for coverage. They were encouraged to "make a crack and sweep the patient toward it." One man describes himself as a former "insurance hit man." He was responsible for recouping money from costly claims by looking for excuses to cancel the policies or by increasing rates for those who racked up large medical bills.

He describes the "prudent-person pre-existing condition" often employed by insurance providers. This clause gives insurers leverage to cancel a policy for a pre-existing condition based on symptoms alone, even if the condition was never diagnosed or treated. A woman who had fallen prey to the prudent-person pre-existing condition had her policy dropped because she had failed to disclose a yeast infection, a "pre-existing condition." Her insurance provider discovered this yeast infection only after her hospital submitted a claim for a surgical procedure. The insurer, rather than paying for the surgery, went through her medical records with a fine-tooth comb, looking for justification to drop her.

A former medical reviewer for a large insurance company used her physician's training to save her company large sums of money by denying claims for lifesaving treatments. She quickly earned a six-figure salary because she was a good medical director in her employer's eyes. She describes the bonus system for medical reviewers: the more denials, the bigger the bonuses. She also confides that the term "medical loss" is insurance industry terminology for a claim that is paid by the insurance company.

Dealing with Refusals

Clearly, the expense of insurance premiums does not guarantee coverage when a patient desperately needs it. How can you avoid the pitfalls of an insurance provider that does not want to provide? Laurie Todd addresses this very issue in *Fight Your Health Insurer and Win*. Her hospital bill totaled $345,000 for lifesaving cancer treatment, including surgery. Because she fought so hard for payment for out-of-network treatment by an out-of-network physician, her insurance provider covered nearly all of it.

Upon discharge from the hospital, Laurie received a bill for $159. She did what any proactive patient would do; she called the hospital and questioned the amount. She found that $150 of that bill was for a private room. Laurie argued that she had not requested a private room. If the hospital does not offer a choice, or if the private room is required by the admitting physician, the patient is not responsible for paying for it. After the hospital agreed to remove that charge, she asked, "Why are you billing me nine dollars?" The billing representative said, "It is because you asked for a glass of juice." Laurie replied, "Well, you got me there. I'll pay the nine dollars." This is why Laurie's nickname is "the insurance warrior"!

Fight Your Health Insurer and Win offers a practical and very thorough approach for appealing an insurance provider's decision. Laurie recommends hitting the insurance company hard and fast with a large package of supporting documentation that refutes any argument they have against the treatment that has been denied. She includes her appeal in her book, with step-by-step instructions for preparation. She recommends hours of research to find supporting documents for the statements in the appeal. For example, a search for peer-reviewed journal articles on a site like PubMed can provide proof that a specialist has no peer for a specific protocol. An online search for the insurer's precedent is also very powerful. An insurer may have paid in the past for a procedure that it now refuses to pay.

Laurie found the name of her insurance provider's CEO by doing an Internet search for the insurance company's name and "CEO" with the current year. Then she did another search with the provider's and CEO's names with "fax" and then "email" to find the CEO's fax number and email address. She found the names of CEOs and medical directors at www.zoominfo.com. She recommends sending an eighty-page fax to the CEO in the middle of the night because it will definitely be noticed the next morning. She refers to her appeal as her War Document. Because she won her war, she is alive and healthy. She bucked the system and refused to listen to her in-network physician who told her that she had two good years left.

Problems with Insurance Plans

Why is all this fighting necessary? Sadly, managed care has shifted the power from physicians to insurance providers. In the online Physician

Survey, respondents cited several difficulties associated with managed care, including lack of time with patients, constraints on testing and treatments for patients, and constraints on referrals to other physicians. Prior to 1973 and the passage of the Health Maintenance Organization Act, physicians had more flexibility in selecting the best options for their patients. Although managed care was intended to contain rising health-care costs while allowing physicians to maintain authority, this movement has evolved into a profitable business for insurance providers (Burton 2009). Now patients and, to a lesser degree, physicians are at the mercy of managed care.

So what exactly is a managed-care plan? What is the difference between an HMO and a PPO? Does anybody get to choose his own doctors anymore? How are we supposed to navigate this confusing labyrinth when we are feeling awful in the first place? If the symptoms don't make us feel bad, the insurance issues certainly will.

A managed-care plan is a health insurance plan that requires or incentivizes an insured person to use providers who are owned or managed by or under contract with the insurer offering the health benefit plan. Managed-care plans differ from traditional health plans, also known as indemnity plans or fee-for-service plans. Traditional health plans allow consumers to select their practitioners and pay for services after a deductible is met. Many traditional plans pay 80 percent of reasonable and customary charges after the deductible is met but before the annual out-of-pocket maximum is met. Once the out-of-pocket maximum is met, many traditional plans will cover 100 percent of the costs.

Managed-care plans cover up to 100 percent of costs if the consumer sees a provider within the network. If the consumer selects an out-of-network provider, the coverage is 60 to 80 percent and sometimes 0 percent. Managed-care plans work well for those who are healthy and those who do not have unusual conditions that require the expertise of out-of-network practitioners. There are three major categories of managed care plans.

- Health maintenance organizations (HMO) cover health-care services when an insured person uses a plan provider. HMOs are generally the most restrictive type of managed care plan and are not as common as PPOs and POSs. HMO coverage is available only for services from a plan provider. The insured person must follow the HMO's procedures for obtaining services, such as obtaining a referral before seeing a specialist and getting pre-authorization for hospitalization or surgery. Limitations on the choice of provider are offset by the lower cost of services.

• Preferred provider organizations (PPO) provide coverage regardless of the choice of provider but generally pay a larger portion of the bill if the insured person uses a provider selected by the plan. PPOs offer greater flexibility than HMOs but have higher out-of-pocket costs for each doctor visit or treatment that is not provided by a preferred provider. This is an option for patients who want more flexibility than an HMO offers but don't need the ultimate flexibility offered by a traditional plan and would like to save money in premiums, deductibles, and co-pays.

• Point-of-service plans (POS) are usually offered by HMOs and provide both HMO-type benefits and traditional health insurance benefits. POS plans provide financial incentives to use network providers but allow insured individuals to choose providers outside the plan. POS plans offer both the flexibility of a traditional plan and the opportunity to save money on co-pays, deductibles, and premiums with an HMO (Belling 2004).

Making Choices About Employer-Provided Insurance

If you receive insurance benefits through your employer, you probably have comparatively low premiums because of the large group rate, cost-sharing from your employer, or both. If you have a choice in selecting a health-care plan, don't allow the costs of premiums to make the decision for you. Look very carefully at your medical situation and that of your family members. What may seem like a bargain on the front end could turn out to be your worst financial nightmare.

The time to look at your health-care options is before accepting the job offer. No matter how lucrative that salary may be, look carefully at the insurance benefits that accompany it. If you are a new college graduate with no income and no health insurance, any plan is better than what you currently have. But if you already have a job and health insurance or if you have several job offers from which to choose, examine your options carefully. If you change jobs and you or a family member has a pre-existing medical condition, check the new employer's insurance provider's pre-existing clause before accepting a job offer.

Once you secure the job, you will sign up for benefits as a new employee. If your new employer has a waiting period before your insurance is effective or before the pre-existing clause expires, make sure you and your family are covered in the interim with COBRA or supplemental insurance. If you have several health-care options, study them carefully and review any questions you have with your employer's benefits representative. Make sure you know what you are selecting because you may have to wait a year to select a different plan. If you or a family member has a rare or chronic condition that requires specialized treatment, you should select the plan that gives you the greatest flexibility in selecting physicians. If you are young and healthy, have no dependents, and are at a lower income level, an HMO might be a better bet because of the lower premiums, co-pays, and deductibles.

Your employer has probably contracted with a very large insurance provider in an effort to get better group rates. If this is the case, you will need help and plenty of ammunition to fight any claims that are denied. Your first line of defense is your employer's benefits representative. She will have a working relationship with the insurance provider's supervisory personnel, and she may have helped resolve for someone else the very problem that you are experiencing. She will know how best to navigate the system and penetrate the layers of red tape that are commonplace among large insurance providers.

If your employer is self-insured, that means the employer rather than the insurer absorbs all costs. Working for a self-insured company is a double-edged sword. On the negative side, the employer has access to your medical information, specifically medical costs incurred by you and your family. On the positive side, you have more leverage fighting to get a medical test or treatment covered. In some cases, the self-insured employer can direct the insurance provider to pay your claim. In other cases, a board composed of corporate benefits professionals and representatives from the insurance provider reviews claims that have been appealed and decides collaboratively whether or not to pay the claim. Your company benefits representative can provide direction on how to appeal a claim in this manner. If you cannot get satisfaction from your benefits representative and if you work for a large corporation, you can voice your concerns to your corporate ombudsman.

Every year, your employer will probably hold open enrollment, the opportunity to change your medical insurance plan. Review your plan carefully to determine whether or not it still works for your situation. If you have a status change (marriage, divorce, birth or death in the immediate family) you should have the option to change your plan during the year, between open enrollments.

When You Don't Have Group Health Insurance

But what if you are not employed, don't have group health insurance, or are retired? If you have lost your job, you probably have the option of selecting COBRA insurance. Under the Consolidated Omnibus Budget Reconciliation Act of 1986 (COBRA), all employers with 20 or more employees must offer former employees and family members continuation of medical coverage at a group rate for up to 18 months. The caveat is that the group rate is the rate that had previously been shared by the employer, plus up to 2 percent for administrative costs. For example, if you had been paying $200 per month for coverage, your rate under COBRA may jump to $408 per month because you will have to absorb your employer's share plus the 2 percent administrative costs. Employers do not have to share premium costs with former employees, although a small number of them do.

If you find yourself in a position to choose COBRA, your number-one priority is pre-existing conditions. If you or a family member has a pre-existing condition, you may have to select COBRA to have that condition covered. Other considerations are medication expenses, ability to qualify for a new insurance plan, pregnancy, or a new job without insurance or with a pre-existing clause.

If you are disabled or retired, you probably have coverage through Medicare. You can learn more about Medicare and supplemental plans at www.medicare.gov. If you qualify for Medicare, you also have the option of selecting a Medicare health plan run by a private company like an HMO or PPO. Keep in mind that you will have the same advantages and disadvantages you would with any HMO or PPO. You will benefit financially if you can stay within the network, but you will not have as much flexibility in selecting your practitioner. On the other hand, if you select the Original Medicare Plan, along with a Medigap plan, your premiums will be higher, but all Medicare-approved claims are paid at nearly 100 percent after a small deductible. And you can choose your medical practitioner; there are no in-network or out-of-network complications. If you qualify for both Medicaid and Medicare, Medicaid may pay your Medicare premiums.

You may encounter some obstacles when trying to find a physician if you are insured through Medicare, Medicaid, or, sadly, Tricare. How unfortunate for those who are struggling; those who have worked their entire lives and paid into Social Security; and those who have served our country only to come home with limited health care. But until our health-care system reaches the level of other industrialized nations, these are the parameters within which we must operate. Contact your local or state medical society to obtain a list of physicians who accept Medicare, Medicaid, or Tricare. You can also visit www.mytricare.com/internet/tric/tri/tricare.nsf or call 1-877-TRICARE (874-2273) to find a physician who accepts Tricare payments.

If you have no medical insurance but can afford monthly premiums, by all means you should make every effort to secure insurance coverage for yourself and your family. You can search your options online at a comprehensive site such as www.ehealthinsurance.com. Your budget may limit you to higher-deductible, lower-premium options, but you will be much better off than with no insurance coverage at all. If you have a number of options and all else is equal, you will have a better chance of appealing denials with a smaller insurer. Smaller insurance providers are more accessible and less likely to be cloaked in bureaucracy than larger ones. Laurie Todd says, "Give me a funky little HMO any time."

Karen Lingar, director of First Community Health Plan, Inc., shares Laurie's sentiment. First Community Health is a small, community-based Medigap plan. As a community health plan, it covers only local in-network hospitals and facilities at the full rate. Consumers can get approval for out-of-network treatment if no other facilities are available (for example, when they are traveling). Sometimes consumers fail to use the right hospital or forget to call during an out-of-town emergency. When they get the bill and call First Community, they have a chance to plead their case. In many instances, First Community relents and pays the claim. What are the chances of a large insurer with annual profits in the billions showing this level of compassion?

Working with Your Insurer

Regardless of your medical insurance plan—group, individual, HMO, PPO, or Medicare—you will face uphill battles while seeking payment of claims by your insurer. But there are ways you can maximize your chances for success.

Maximizing Your Chances for Success with Insurance

Study your insurance plan thoroughly. Your insurer publishes a booklet or directory each year that details which services are covered. Eligible services can change from one year to the next. Know what is covered before you seek treatment. Make sure you are clear on all pre-authorization requirements for procedures and hospitalizations.

Appeal denied claims quickly. Some insurers allow only a 60-day window for appeals.

Read EOBs (explanation of benefits) quickly and thoroughly. The more quickly you catch a problem, the better. Keep a file with EOBs and billing statements from your doctors. If you have Medicare, you will probably receive the doctor bill for a denied claim much more quickly than your EOB, also known as the Medicare Summary Statement. Medicare issues this statement quarterly unless you request otherwise.

Keep EOBs for at least a year, longer if you have incurred a lot of medical expenses. I have received bills from physicians' offices more than a year after the date of service. I was grateful for the dated EOB that explained why my insurer had not paid the claim.

Question charges. Try to resist the urge to pay a balance you don't understand just to get your doctor's office or the hospital billing department off your back. Better yet, ask the billing person to refile the claim if you suspect it was not filed properly. On several occasions, I have been billed because my secondary insurance was billed before the primary insurance. Question both the medical provider and your insurance provider to determine where the problem lies.

Ask your medical provider, particularly a hospital, for an itemized bill. You may be surprised at the charges for treatments and services that you did not receive. Bogus charges are probably the result of a billing error, but they are sometimes attributed to cost shifting. This practice forces insured patients to absorb the charges for uninsured patients.

Exhaust your insurance provider's appeal process. You will be required to do this before your state insurance commissioner will agree to help. To avoid a lengthy appeal process, make sure you include all pertinent information the first time, including the date of service, name of provider, claim number, and circumstances. And as both Laurie Todd and Karen Lingar suggest, provide plenty of supporting information the insurer does not already have. If you offer mounds of irrefutable evidence on the first appeal, you are less likely to need a second appeal. You have the right to request an independent medical review of your case.

These options are helpful for people with medical insurance. But what if you don't have insurance and cannot afford the premiums? You have a number of other options.

If You Don't Have Insurance...

Find out if you qualify for Medicaid. For more information on Medicaid, visit www.cms.hhs.gov/home/medicaid.asp. If you qualify, Medicaid will pay for medical care and prescriptions and will even cover expenses retroactively for three months prior to the application. Many hospitals offer an information packet on Medicaid to patients who cannot pay their hospital bills. You can find out if you qualify for Medicaid or other state or federal programs at www.govbenefits.gov/govbenefits_en.portal or www.benefitscheckup.org.

Seek help at a facility covered under the Hill-Burton Act of 1946. Hospitals, nursing homes, and other health-care facilities obligated under the Hill-Burton Act must offer free or reduced care to patients with incomes at or below the U.S. Department of Health & Human Services poverty guidelines (http://aspe.hhs.gov/poverty/09poverty.shtml). Patients with income up to two times the poverty guidelines may be eligible for treatment at a Hill-Burton facility. For a list of these facilities, visit www.hrsa.gov/hillburton/hillburtonfacilities.htm or call the Hill Burton Hotline at 1-800-638-0742 (1-800-492-0359 in Maryland).

Ask for help at the hospital. Many hospitals offer a packet of information at the registration desk that includes local resources for free and reduced care. Hospitals also employ case managers or social workers who can help you find free or reduced-cost health-care options and also work out a payment plan in the event that you need emergency care at the hospital. Nonprofit hospitals with thriving foundations often provide indigent care and write off the expenses.

Ask for a group rate. Hospitals and physicians often discount their fees to insured patients, so insurance companies are billed at a lower rate, sometimes cut in half. You may be able to negotiate a lower rate with hospitals and doctors, along with a payment plan. A bill totaling thousands of dollars can be negotiated down to hundreds, in many cases.

Find a federally funded community clinic in your area. Federally funded community clinics and look-alike clinics (they function the same but don't have federal funding) must comply with federal regulations and their own plan as described in their grant requests. They offer inexpensive medical care to the uninsured and underinsured, and they accept Medicare and Medicaid. You can search for a federally funded clinic in your community at findahealthcenter.hrsa.gov, or call 1-888-ASK-HRSA (275-4772).

Seek out privately funded, free, or reduced-cost clinics in your community. If a federally funded or look-alike clinic is adequate for the community, it may be the only option for those who are uninsured or underinsured. But for larger communities, the need arises for additional resources, and privately funded clinics open up. Some of them offer free health care to those without private insurance, Medicare, or Medicaid. Others offer lower-cost services. You can find out if your community has these options by checking with your department of human resources or your county health department, or by dialing 211, a nationwide service that provides information on human services. Your housing authority will probably have information on local human services, including free or reduced-cost medical care.

Find out if your community has a Project Access program. You can check with your hospital or the services listed above, or search online by entering "Project Access medical" in your Web browser. This is not a nationwide service, but many cities are modeling it after existing programs in other cities. To find out how Project Access works, visit www.pbcms.org/index.cfm?fuseaction=pages.projectaccess for information on the Palm Beach County program.

Project Access is a collaborative effort between physicians, diagnostic centers, hospitals, and pharmacies to provide free medical care to patients who qualify, usually those under a specified income with no private insurance and no government assistance. The program is vital to those who need hospitalization, screening procedures, or surgery. A hospital emergency department cannot turn anybody away, but a hospital can refuse nonemergency treatment to a patient who cannot be pre-authorized with private insurance, Medicare, or Medicaid. If you are above the income level to qualify for Medicaid and you cannot afford insurance, Project Access is your best hope for obtaining services such as nonemergency surgery or diagnostic tests such as colonoscopy.

Take advantage of free or reduced-cost screenings. Health fairs are great opportunities for free or reduced-cost screenings. You may also find state or local programs that offer medical screening assistance for uninsured or underinsured patients. The Breast Cancer Relief Foundation has partnered with several major hospitals for breast cancer screening assistance. For more information, visit www.breastcancerrelief.org/preventionEarlyDetection.asp. Check with your hospital, department of human resources, or county health department, or dial 211 to find out which programs are available in your community.

Take advantage of county health department services. County health departments offer free services including immunizations and health education; HIV and sexually transmitted disease counseling, diagnosis and treatment; tuberculosis testing, and WIC (Women, Infants and Children). Birth control treatment is available at a reduced cost on a sliding scale, based on income. WIC provides health assessments, education, and supplemental food to pregnant and postpartum women, infants, and children up to age five. The USDA's Food and Nutrition Service also offers information at www.fns.usda.gov/wic.

Use special programs for children. Every state offers free or reduced-cost medical insurance to children under the age of nineteen who qualify. To learn more about your state's program, visit www.insurekidsnow.gov, or call 1-877-KIDS-NOW (543-7669). Some states and communities have programs for children who do not qualify for Medicaid or the state program. You can call 211 to find out what is offered locally or statewide. A number of communities have school-based health services available free or at a reduced cost for children who do not qualify for state or federal services. Your county or city board of education will have that information.

Know your rights as a veteran. For health benefits information, visit wwwl.va.gov/health/index.asp or call 1-800-827-1000. With the introduction of Project Hero in 2005 (www.va.gov/hac/hero/objectives. asp), veterans have better access to more expedient treatment. You can also contact your state VA office, or a local veteran's advocacy group may be available to help you navigate the complexities of the VA health insurance system.

Contact your area agency on aging if you are a senior citizen. You may qualify for local or state programs created to help senior citizens with health-care costs. For more information, visit www.n4a.org. And by all means, check with your senior center for free or reduced services, including medication counseling, screenings, and immunizations.

Protect your mental health. If you suffer from a chronic condition or have developed a life-threatening illness, you and your family may benefit from mental health counseling. Inexpensive treatment is available on a sliding-scale basis at local mental health centers. To access a listing of resources in your area, visit mentalhealth.samhsa.gov. For family counseling associated with a terminal illness, contact your hospice provider. Hospice provides not only patient care, but also spiritual and emotional care for the entire family. Most hospice organizations are funded through private donations and Medicare. If you have insurance coverage, you can expect mental health coverage that aligns closely with coverage of physical illness, thanks to passage of the Mental Health Parity Bill in 2009.

Making a Difference

Our health-care system does not present a pretty picture. There are no easy answers, and there is no quick fix for what ails it. Unfortunately, our two-trillion-dollar health-care system is at the center of a fierce war with four armies battling for control: health insurers, hospitals, government and, to a lesser degree, physicians. The physicians, whose interests are most closely aligned with those of patients, are losing the war, according to Regina Herzlinger, author of the best-selling book *Who Killed Health-care?* She advocates a health-care system controlled by consumers and physicians and calls readers to action (quoted in Announcing 2007).

We need a health-care system that makes medical care available to everyone regardless of income level. A nation as sophisticated as ours should not tolerate the shameful practice of patient dumping or allow patients to die on the hospital floor while awaiting treatment. Our challenge is in making health-care available to everyone without cutting the salaries of some of the lower-paid professionals, particularly primary care physicians and nurses. We are already short of both, and the system will not survive additional shortages.

Although the transition to a more functional system will take time, there are things that we can do individually to make a difference collectively. As individuals, we can reduce some of the unnecessary spending on medical costs by practicing preventive care (see chapters 2 and 3), ensuring the right treatment for the right condition with proactive patient behavior, and coordinating efforts among multiple doctors to avoid redundant tests and treatments. We can be a part of the solution.

Chapter 8

"Someone Took Away Our Swords," Part Two

Dealing with drug/dental/vision coverage, disability, and workers' compensation

Medical insurance coverage is woefully inadequate for many people, but prescription, dental, and vision coverage is even worse. A number of health-insurance plans do not cover these areas adequately, if at all. Thus, prescription, dental, and vision expenses are treated as luxuries in some households.

One consolation is the fact that these expenses, along with other out-of-pocket medical expenses, may be tax-deductible. If your out-of-pocket medical expenses are more than 7.5 percent of your adjusted gross income, you can deduct the amount of medical and dental expenses *over* that limit. (For a listing of includible medical expenses, visit www.irs.gov/publications/p502/ar02.html#en_US_publink100014783.)

After surveying free and low-cost options for those without adequate coverage in these areas, this chapter advises you on dealing with disability-insurance claims, Social Security disability, and workers' compensation.

Dealing with Prescription Coverage

If you have generous prescription coverage, consider yourself blessed. Prescription coverage is a hot topic, especially among those who have Medicare Part D. Most Medicare Part D plans cover medications at 75 percent after the deductible (zero to $295, depending on the plan) is met. The plan covers medication at 75 percent until the consumer has incurred a total of $2700 in actual retail drug costs for the year. At that point, the plan invokes the dreaded "donut hole." During the donut hole phase, the consumer pays for medications at 100 percent until he has spent a total of $4350 out of pocket during the year. Then the plan pays for medications at 95 percent for the rest of the year, and the entire process starts over on January 1. The problem is that most people do not reach the catastrophic level at which the plan pays 95 percent of the drug costs. The average Medicare consumer spends two thousand dollars annually in out-of-pocket medication costs according to the movie *Sicko*.

If you do not have adequate prescription coverage, you may be able to save on prescriptions costs with one of the following resources:

- *Comprehensive sites for prescription-assistance programs.* Visit a Web site that has compiled comprehensive information on free or reduced-cost prescriptions. Partnership for Prescription Assistance provides information for over 450 programs with more than 180 participating pharmaceutical companies. For more information, visit www.pparx.org or call 1-888-477-2669. One pharmaceutical provider, Pfizer, recently launched a new program that provides free medication for up to one year to newly unemployed consumers who qualify. For more information, call 1-866-706-2400, or visit www.pfizerhelpfulanswers.com/pages/misc/Default.aspx. Together Access RX offers savings of 25 to 40 percent to patients without prescription insurance. Learn more at www.togetherrx access.com/Tx/jsp/home.jsp or by calling 1-800-444-4106. You can also visit www.rxassist.org, click on the Patients section, and search the database, or call 401-729-3284 for a program that might help you.

- *Federally funded and privately funded clinics.* They may offer free or reduced-cost prescriptions. To find federally funded clinics, visit findahealthcenter.hrsa.gov, or call 1-888-ASK-HRSA (275-4772). You can also find privately funded clinics by contacting the local health department or department of human resources or by calling 211.

- *Project Access, if it is available and if you qualify.* Project Access programs often include free or reduced-cost medication.

- *Online discount coupons.* You can find free, downloadable discount coupons for medications at www.internetdrugcoupons .com.

- *Free samples.* Be honest with your physician and tell her that you cannot afford your medication. She may have free samples she can give you.

- *Generic or alternative treatments.* If your physician does not have free samples to offer, ask if there is an alternative treatment or a generic alternative.

Options for Optical and Dental Care

As if prescription costs aren't enough to worry about, what about optical and dental care? Many employers offer dental insurance, but many do not offer insurance for optical care. However, most employers offer an option that allows employees to put money into a tax-free account to use for out-of-pocket expenses such as optical care. You should consider this option if your family uses optical or other noncovered services frequently. Your medical insurance may cover optical exams if your visual problems are related to a medical cause such as diabetes. Your medical insurance may also cover screenings for diseases such as macular degeneration or retinitis pigmentosa if you have a strong family history. To find out if you qualify for free or reduced-cost optical care, visit:

- Access to Care at www.eyecareamerica.org/eyecare/care, or call 1-800-222-3937

- Vision USA at www.aoa.org/visionusa.xml, or call 1-800-766-4466

- Lions Eye Health Program at www.lionsclubs.org/EN/content/lcif_gr_lehp.shtml, or call 630-571-5466

If you don't have dental insurance, your best bet is to avoid dental expenses by using good, consistent oral hygiene habits. Brushing, flossing, and regular cleanings can save you money in the long run by preventing not just dental, but possibly medical problems too. If you drink bottled water, your teeth are not getting adequate fluoride from water. You will need a toothpaste with fluoride, and this is especially important for children to prevent tooth decay. Private dental insurance is available, but it rarely yields any savings for patients in the long run. There are a few programs that may be helpful to people without dental insurance who qualify:

- The U.S. Department of Health & Human Services offers two possible avenues. For a list of dental reimbursement program clinics, visit hab.hrsa.gov/programs/dentallist.htm. To find federally funded clinics, visit findahealthcenter.hrsa.gov.

- Privately funded clinics that offer free or reduced-cost care may also offer dental care. Call 211 or your local health department or Department of Human Resources to find out if your community has such a clinic.

- Dental schools provide quality, low-cost care. Visit www.nidcr.nih .gov/FindingDentalCare, or call the National Oral Health Information Clearinghouse at (301) 402–7364 to find the dental school nearest you.

- If you have Medicaid, visit www.cms.hhs.gov/MedicaidDentalCoverage to find out if you are eligible for dental coverage.

- Children under nineteen years of age are eligible for dental care under your state's medical program at www.insurekidsnow.gov or 1-877-KIDS-NOW (543-7669).

- Your community or state may have other dental assistance programs. Call 211 for more information or check with your United Way agency.

Disability and Workers' Compensation

Lightning and electric shock survivors who are fortunate enough to have medical insurance usually obtain it through Medicare via Social Security disability or workers' compensation. If they make it through the process of fighting for one of these benefits, they have made it through the worst part of the storm. Some don't make it and commit suicide in the midst of this emotionally draining process. I'll never forget one of our annual conferences, where our president and founder, Steve Marshburn, announced that he and other board members had talked eleven LS&ESSI members out of suicide the previous year.

Because of fraudulent applications for disability and workers' compensation, the system must weed out the malingerers, unfortunately resulting in a process that is degrading to those who really are suffering. The true sufferers must endure harsh treatment from those who are tasked with denying applicants who do not meet strict criteria. Applicants for workers' compensation tell horror stories of being stalked by private investigators their insurance companies hired in an attempt to catch them doing some kind of "nondisabled" activity. The problem is that disability is not black and white. What looks like a nondisabled activity may render the person incapacitated for the next several days.

Joe and Cheryll's Story

I met Joe and his wife, Cheryll, during an LS&ESSI conference and was impressed by their strength and the way they fought their battle so synergistically. Joe had become disabled after a lightning injury that occurred on the job. He applied for Social Security disability and fared better than most applicants, receiving a favorable decision within several months. The Social Security Administration (SSA) awarded him back pay for the time he had waited for a decision, a lump sum payment. Fortunately, Joe and Cheryll did not spend that money. Ten months later, the SSA notified Joe that he had been overpaid and instructed him to return $18,000 within 30 days—at Christmastime.

The disability income, approximately one-third of Joe's former income, helped him and his family while they waited for approval for workers' compensation. Because Joe had witnesses to his on-the-job injury, he did not anticipate a problem. However, what followed was a nightmarish five-year series of doctor visits, including at least half a dozen psychiatric evaluations ordered by the Bureau of Workers' Compensation. To further compound the situation, Joe's major symptoms were not always visible. He had severe pain throughout his entire body and debilitating fatigue. He also had sporadic seizures and myoclonic jerks, the only visible indication of a physical problem.

Joe and Cheryll endured one physical evaluation after another and numerous hearings. During one evaluation, Joe was subjected to rigorous testing designed to prove that he was not disabled. He was ordered to walk, crawl, carry drywall, and work puzzles for two hours to determine whether or not he could work an eight-hour day. He became so agitated that he tried harder to accomplish the tasks, a move that did not work in his favor. The evaluator prepared a report indicating that Joe was indeed able to work full-time despite the fact that this two-hour ordeal rendered him bedridden for a week.

Just prior to his final hearing before a workers' compensation judge, Joe was hospitalized for his condition. He was visibly weak and had uncontrollable hand movements when he appeared before the judge. Joe was fortunate to have an understanding physician who went to the disability hearing on his behalf. His condition, his physician, and the 75 pages that Cheryll had faxed to his attorney helped him finally receive a favorable decision after a grueling five-year battle. That's right—Joe and Cheryll had an attorney helping them through this nightmare. Imagine what they would have faced without one!

But the story does not end there. Although Joe was declared permanently and totally disabled and although workers' compensation is supposed to cover the cost of his medications, Joe and Cheryll have to fight and appeal on a regular basis to get the prescription coverage to which he is entitled. They have dealt with the secondary issues of insurance, disability, and workers' compensation while mourning the loss of their old lives and while Joe suffers with the physical symptoms of his injury.

Many Challenges to Face

As you can see, the battle for disability or workers' compensation is nearly impossible to fight alone. At the very least, you need a great support system, and in many cases, an attorney can make a huge difference. Disability and workers' compensation attorneys are typically paid on a percentage basis and only if the decision is favorable. It is money well spent.

The workers' compensation process varies from one state to another. Some states are lawsuit states, and others hear cases before an administrative law judge. If you experience an on-the-job injury, you must report the injury to your supervisor as soon as possible. If you do not report your injury in a timely fashion (within thirty days in most states), you not only risk losing benefits, but you put your employer in jeopardy with oversight agencies such as OSHA (Occupational Health and Safety Administration) and NIOSH (National Institute for Occupational Safety and Health).

You need a medical certification to file a claim with your employer's insurer, and you will be required to see the physician of your employer's choice, usually a physician contracted by the employer. The fairness of workers' compensation agency physicians also varies from one to another. The agency physician's job is to treat the patient but at the same time try and reduce the amount of compensation awarded. After the initial assessment by the employer's physician, you can then include your own physicians in the panel that will make a determination.

In most states, the employer's insurance provider pays the workers' compensation benefits to the employee after the employer has submitted a report to the insurance provider and the state workers' compensation board or industrial commission. If the insurance provider rejects the claim and refuses to pay workers' compensation benefits, the employee can pursue arbitration with the state workers' compensation board or industrial commission. If the employee is not successful with arbitration, he can pursue a series of appeals, as Joe did during his pursuit for workers' compensation benefits (Moore 2009).

Your biggest challenge will be proving that an on-the-job injury caused all of the symptoms you are having. Unfortunately, symptoms don't always appear right away. The insurance carrier must be certain that your symptoms occurred as a result of the accident before it will approve workers' compensation benefits. The insurer may look for any possible evidence that your symptoms predated the accident and that you have a pre-existing condition, not a valid workers' compensation case. It will probably deny your case if you do not report the accident quickly. If you are denied benefits after the initial physician certification, you should hire a worker's compensation attorney right away.

You may receive an offer to settle for a lump sum, but give plenty of thought to that decision. Make sure that the amount will be enough for you and your family to live on for the rest of your life. You should also discuss any lump sum offer with a financial advisor and your attorney before making a decision.

The workers' compensation process has its imperfections, as Charles Blevins, OTA, MS, and Daniel Valdez, MD, contend in their book *Solving the Workers' Compensation Puzzle*. They discuss the various participants—the employer, the health-care provider(s), the rehabilitation provider(s), the insurer, the insurance adjuster, the case manager/rehabilitation nurse, the pre-authorization physician or nurse, the impairment physician, the medical auditor, the injured employee, and the attorney—all with different agendas. No wonder the process is so daunting! (Blevins 2007, 19-38).

Qualifying for Disability

If you become disabled and if you qualify for Social Security disability, you can expect to receive approximately one-third of your previous salary. In a best-case scenario, you will have to lower your standard of living by two-thirds unless you have another source of income.

If you become disabled and have disability insurance (most likely through an employer), you can apply for disability compensation. If approved, you can expect to receive around two-thirds of your previous income. Unfortunately, you will face a tougher battle trying to qualify for disability through your insurance provider than through Social Security. Insurance companies don't like to pay unless they are absolutely sure that a claimant is disabled. If you don't have a clear-cut diagnosis, you will have an especially difficult time proving a disability to an insurance company, even more so than with Social Security. If you are turned down by your disability-insurance company, that is not the end. You can and should appeal the unfavorable decision if you are covered under a group plan. If not, you will need to exhaust all nonjudicial actions required by the policy before you file a lawsuit against the company.

You can apply simultaneously for Social Security disability and for disability insurance through an insurance provider. In fact, a favorable Social Security decision may give you more credibility with the insurance provider. However, both are very difficult to obtain. If you are successful in securing both Social Security disability and disability compensation from your insurer, you will be subject to an offset or a reduction in disability insurance proceeds. Workers' compensation operates the same way; it offsets disability compensation.

The Social Security disability application process is a particularly laborious one. The SSA sets federal guidelines but contracts with each state for disability determination. The state disability examiners have some leeway in decisions but must follow federal guidelines. You can find an outline of the steps of the process at the end of this chapter.

If you file a workers' compensation claim, a disability claim, or apply for Social Security disability, be prepared for a long and difficult battle like the ones that Joe and Cheryll endured. But a workers' compensation battle, like a disability or Social Security disability battle, is well worth the effort. Not only will you acquire the compensation that you need and deserve, but you will have the satisfaction of knowing that you fought the battle valiantly and unarmed.

It may seem unfair that you have fight so hard for such basics as medical insurance, prescription coverage, disability, and worker's compensation while also struggling with debilitating symptoms. These battles, combined with the fight for a correct diagnosis, can make a disability a full-time job. Although it is a job you would prefer not to have, it may be the most important one you will ever have. Keep in mind especially that one of your most important duties is delegation—you cannot do it alone. You must "rally the troops" and ask for help. You need a strong support system to fight these battles. You may have to fight unarmed, but you do not have to fight alone.

The Process of Applying for Social Security Disability

1. You complete the initial claim. The best way to tackle the paperwork is online. This option gives you time to find names of medications and names and addresses of physicians and is much better than meeting with a rushed claims representative. Be sure to offer complete addresses and phone numbers of physicians so that the disability determination office can procure your medical records as quickly as possible. The process is slow enough as it is; you don't need to create further delays.

2. The claims representative sends your paperwork to the disability determination office. Once the disability determination office has received your claim, it will send you a very long questionnaire that asks penetrating questions about your daily living activities. The disability determination office will also include additional questionnaires to be completed by someone who lives with you and someone who lives outside the home. When completing the questionnaire, be as specific as possible. Don't exaggerate your condition, but don't put a positive spin on it, either. Now is not the time to look like a hero. Describe the realities of your condition in a way that allows the disability examiner to feel your symptoms.

3. The disability examiner reviews your claim and issues a decision. You will receive the decision about six months after the initial application. Unless you have a presumptive disability, you will probably be denied disability compensation. Presumptive disability is a condition that is without any doubt disabling, such as terminal cancer, end-stage renal failure, or advanced AIDS. Eighty-nine percent of claims are denied at this stage. This seems harsh, but if every claim were approved, there would not be enough money for everyone. Disability examiners have to represent the claimants and the taxpayers, and they must be as objective as possible. If you are denied and do not already have an attorney, you should find one who specializes in disability cases. Most disability attorneys also handle workers' compensation cases.

4. Your attorney files an appeal. After the appeal is filed, you will be scheduled to appear before an administrative law judge. Your hearing date will be 283 to 943 days after your attorney has filed the appeal. Your hearing will probably take place before an administrative law judge, but in some cases, hearings are held using live video feed, so you may not even get to see the judge in person. In video hearings especially, you should wear muted colors and little or no jewelry. Your goal is to keep the focus on you and eliminate distractions. Your attorney will offer tips on how to present yourself either in person or on video. Although your attorney is not allowed to coach you, he will give you an idea of the questions you can expect and what kind of information you need to report.

5. *The administrative law judge makes a decision.* Hopefully, you will receive a favorable decision. If so, you will receive a lump sum of disability compensation retroactive to the date of your disability, and your monthly compensation will begin. Keep in mind that the lump sum is not all yours to keep. You can be taxed on up to 85 percent of your disability compensation, and your attorney will receive a percentage, with a ceiling of $6000. You will be eligible for Medicare coverage two years after the month in which you became disabled.

6. *You can pursue additional appeals.* If you receive an unfavorable decision, you can appeal to the Social Security Appeals Council, which will hear your case within twelve to twenty-four months. If your appeal is not successful, the next step is the first one outside the SSA. You can file a lawsuit with the U.S. District Court. If you are still not successful, you can appeal to the Circuit Court and then to the Supreme Court. With each appeal, your chances for a favorable decision improve. The last two steps are rare. Most claimants either receive a favorable decision earlier in the process or are told by their attorneys that they do not have a case.

7. *Expect ongoing reviews.* Once you are receiving compensation, the disability determination office schedules regular reviews to determine whether or not your status has changed. The frequency of reviews

depends on your level of disability. There are three levels of disability: 1) improvement expected, 2) improvement possible, and 3) no improvement expected. For level 1, reviews are conducted every one to two years; for level 2, every three to four years, and for level 3, every five to seven years.

If you improve enough to resume employment, you can use the Ticket to Work program and other incentives. You may have a trial work period of nine months during which you can make sure you are able to work. During this time, you will retain disability compensation while earning employment income. After the trial work period, you can earn up to $980 per month without losing disability compensation for that month. If your income is under $700 per month, you will not be subject to the trial work period.

Part 2:

Taking Charge of Your Attitude

Chapter 9

"Find Happiness Wherever You Can"

Managing Adversity and Seeing Its Gifts

Five years ago, I was the chairperson of the Huntsville Area Committee on Employment of People with Disabilities. Our board was planning its annual awards banquet to honor employees with disabilities and professionals and organizations that promote employment opportunities for them. Every year, we had been blessed with powerful, inspirational guest speakers. One woman shared her remarkable story as a survivor of one of the U.S. Embassy bombings in Kenya. Another speaker shared his poignant experiences as the father of a woman battling schizophrenia. All of our amazing guest speakers had elicited powerful emotions from the audience, resulting in standing ovations. Because we had set the bar so high, I was worried. *How will we find yet another extraordinary speaker this year?*

A fellow board member suggested that I contact Milton Anthony, a man who had survived a bombing that left him blind, mostly deaf, and a triple amputee. I contacted Milton and made the arrangements for him to speak at our banquet. During our telephone conversations, I thought, *This guy is a hoot!* Milton did not disappoint. His presentation brought the audience to tears and laughter and drew a rousing standing ovation. When I approached him after the banquet, he was wrapping up a conversation with a man who said, "I'll see you later." Milton quipped, "You'll see me before I see you!" I was in awe of his strength, his humor, and his natural gift for putting others at ease with his disabilities.

When seeking interviewees for this book, I immediately thought of

Milton and his insight on adversity and strength. During our two-and-a-half-hour interview, his effusive, animated demeanor was infectious, and he had me laughing to the point of tears. Without thinking, I said, "You should do stand-up comedy," and he chuckled and replied, "Yeah, but I can't stand up for very long!" It wasn't what he said, but the way he said it that was so comical. With his sunny disposition, this man could cheer up the grumpiest of the grumpy. He looks for the joy in everything.

Milton had lived a healthy but dangerous life before the accident that disabled him. He was a member of an international motorcycle club that often sparred with other clubs. He'd been attracted to the motorcycle gang life from an early age, seduced by feelings of power and invincibility. Each time he cheated death, he fed that invincibility. He'd had four opportunities when rival gangs made attempts on his life. The fifth attempt was nearly successful. Milton received a phone call asking him to meet a member of a rival gang behind a bar for negotiations to "stop the bloodshed." There, he saw a beautiful hand-painted Harley-Davidson motorcycle gas tank sitting on top of a concrete block. Thinking that it must be some kind of a peace offering, he picked it up.

Three and a half weeks later, Milton regained consciousness in the hospital. What he had thought was a peace offering turned out to be a sophisticated and deadly bomb. The gas tank contained six sticks of dynamite and had blown him 75 feet across the parking lot. When his wife initially saw him in the hospital, she would not have known it was him had it not been for an identifying childhood scar. Because of the morphine and hallucinations, Milton did not realize for several days that he had lost his sight and most of his hearing. As he was trying to grasp that horrible reality, he spent 16 hours over a five-day period undergoing amputations of part of his leg, part of one arm, and part of one hand. He was hit with all of these losses more quickly than he could absorb what was happening to him, and excruciating phantom pain started after his hospitalization.

As Milton struggled to adjust to his new and very different life, he regained 40 percent of his hearing with the use of a hearing aid. Before he got the hearing aid, he found it nearly impossible to navigate even a simple walk from one room to another. Not only did he have to adjust to his prosthetic leg, but he could not follow another person because he could not hear that person's voice. Milton eventually learned to adapt to his new challenges with the help of his wife and his motorcycle club brothers.

Unfortunately, his marriage crumbled under the strain of his multiple disabilities, and he suddenly found himself alone, angry, and frustrated because he was unable to take care of himself. But out of that frustration came a new resolve, and Milton vowed never to become dependent upon another person ever again. He learned to do everything for himself— cooking, cleaning, laundry, and shopping. During the next eight years, he earned his GED and then bachelor's and master's degrees. He created and sold voice-recognition software for visually impaired consumers. He earned a counseling license, and today he counsels people dealing with adversity and teaches pain-management classes. He is a public speaker and is writing his memoirs, using voice-recognition software.

As you can see, happiness is not only possible in spite of adversity; in some cases, happiness is possible *because of* adversity. Milton's life is much more fulfilling than it was before the bombing. He no longer takes the beauty of life for granted. He is happily remarried to a wonderful woman named Linda, and he has enriched her life as much as she has enriched his. He has provided her with a sense of adventure that she had never known. She has been a great source of strength and support for him, but only to the extent that he will allow. Because of his vow never again to be dependent upon another person, Milton allows her to help him only when he requests that help.

How can someone with such debilitating injuries find such peace and happiness? Milton not only conveys happiness, he is downright exuberant in every conversation and e-mail. How is this possible?

My Experience of Choosing Happiness

Happiness is a choice and a responsibility. During my nine-year period of disability, a wise psychotherapist advised me to "find happiness wherever you can." His simple but profound statement resonated deeply with me and became my mantra. His advice forced me to take responsibility for my own happiness and not to impose that responsibility on the physicians whom I hoped would properly diagnose and cure me. He was respectful and compassionate, but he held me accountable for my own emotional well-being.

I found that I had to work much harder at finding and creating my own happiness while disabled. And because of my limitations, I found happiness in some of the simplest things. When I was at my lowest functioning level, one of my drivers helped me navigate around a bookstore. I was able to stay in the store just long enough to select a couple of mystery books and buy a cappuccino before the stimuli created by all of the books placed close together became too much for my brain to process. On the way back to the car, I was absolutely elated and said, "I have a coffee drink and mystery books. Life doesn't get any better than this!" My driver replied, "Wow, it doesn't take much to make you happy!" She could not possibly have known how much that visit to the bookstore meant to me. I'd been unable to go anywhere or do anything, and that experience was pure heaven.

Finding New Pursuits

My disability gave me opportunities for a number of creative pursuits. I learned to use a hot-glue gun and make wreaths, ornaments, and flower arrangements. I baked homemade cookies and gave them as gifts for Christmas. I learned to use Adobe Photoshop and Illustrator and started a small greeting card business. My drivers took me around to sell cards and even T-shirts in gift shops. I didn't make a profit, but I had fun and, more important, a sense of purpose. I found the phone and Internet invaluable in staying connected with the outside world. With Joe's business travel, I often went four or five days at a stretch with no human contact. When my symptoms were at their very worst, I had great difficulty in walking two houses down the street to visit a neighbor. But as unusual as my existence was, I could be like anyone else online. The Internet leveled the playing field.

Finding Companions

While dealing with mysterious, undiagnosed symptoms, I also battled flare-ups of ulcerative colitis from time to time. I joined a local Crohn's and Colitis Support Group and found comfort for not only the colitis but the other symptoms as well. Because I was unable to drive, I rode to the meetings with two women who lived nearby, both named Linda. After one of the meetings, I confided to both Lindas that my driver was planning to stop working for the assisted-living service that I was using and that I needed a new driver. One of them expressed interest in taking over as my driver. She wanted to earn some extra income but did not want to leave her 15-month-old son, Mitchell, in day care. She saw the arrangement as a way to keep him with her while working. We agreed to give it a try and see how it worked out.

During our first outing, we discovered some uncanny connections. We have the same birthday, and we're both daughters of educators, the only girl in the family, and the middle child. During subsequent outings, we found that we have the same IQ and are the only people in Alabama who don't like iced tea! We share very similar beliefs, ethics, and political views. We knew right away that God had brought us together for a reason.

During the next five and a half years, our friendship grew, and Linda, Mitchell, and I became like family. We went out twice a week for four to five hours so I could get my errands done. When I was at my worst and could not get groceries, Linda got them for me. I gave her my list and debit card, and she knew instinctively what to select if the item of my choice was not available. Although she was there to help, she made sure that my condition did not define me. We laughed and joked from the time we left my house until we returned.

Linda and I had opportunities to help each other cope with the loss of our beloved pets (Brandy and Sheba passed away during this time), and we helped each other pick up the pieces as both of our marriages crumbled. We offered each other support during health crises that occurred along the way. We would not have had this opportunity had it not been for my disability. Because of it, Linda and Mitchell have become my surrogate sister and nephew. Adversity gives us gifts we would not have experienced otherwise.

The Gifts of Adversity

My disability also provided the gifts of spiritual growth, personal growth, and strength. My relationship with God was strengthened as I sought His help and His wisdom. I grew as a person and learned to appreciate both the simple things in life and the important things in life. I found that when we have our health, we do indeed have everything. Without good health, we cannot enjoy or even manage the things that we often put ahead of it, such as family and careers. We tend to take our health for granted until something goes wrong. Health is like anything else—we don't realize what we have until it is gone.

I gained insight into human nature. Support from friends and family showed me the true beauty of the human spirit. They were kind, compassionate, and desperate to help me find answers. But I had to make an effort to reach out to others to maintain relationships. Because I was isolated by my circumstances, I had to work hard to keep the world from passing me by. But today, I am grateful for the circumstances that pushed me out of my comfort zone. I learned to take the initiative to tell others what I need and ask for help, which was very difficult. Sometimes, God gives us experiences we need but don't necessarily want.

The most enduring gift my disability provided is strength. With strength comes confidence, and I know now that I can handle anything life throws my way. I would not be the person I am today had I not experienced this taxing but amazing odyssey. Based on my journey, I doubt that strength is possible without first experiencing adversity. Cheri Cowell, author of *Direction: Discernment for the Decisions of Your Life* agrees that adversity is necessary for personal growth and an important part of human life. Cowell asserts that adversity is a gift if we use it as such—not an easy task when we are in the throes of a crisis. Yes, hardship builds character, but we would all rather do without it.

Adversity's gifts all sound very nice, bordering on Pollyannaish, but what if you just plain feel bad and don't want to be positive? That is okay. You certainly have every right to be angry if a big part of your life has been taken away. It is okay to be angry with God—He can take it. When you have lost a part of yourself, you can expect to experience the stages of grief: disbelief, yearning, anger, depression, and acceptance (Meek 2007). There is no way around grief, you must go through it and allow yourself to feel the emotions that accompany it. Give in to the emotions, but don't let them consume you. Indulge your anger, but set a time limit on it. Feel free to throw yourself a pity party once in a while. The best way to feel validated is by validating yourself.

Embracing Your New Life

If you are suffering from a debilitating medical condition or injury, try to resist the tendency to turn your anger inward and to feel guilty or beat yourself up emotionally. You are not to blame, and you have no reason to feel guilty. You are one of God's children, created in His image and loved by Him to the same extent as any of His children. You are still the amazing person you have always been. You just have a different life now. That doesn't mean it has to be a less rewarding life. Keep in mind that Milton Anthony's life became more fulfilling after the accident that claimed his sight, most of his hearing, and three of his extremities. You can embrace your new life and find strengths and gifts you didn't know you had. Your life may not be the one you had envisioned, but when life throws you a curve, sometimes the best thing you can do is follow it. Fighting the inevitable is a waste of energy that you need for other endeavors.

That is not to say that you should give up and just accept your circumstances. If there is a chance that you can improve your physical condition, by all means, keep fighting and don't stop looking for answers. But at the same time, you must accept the circumstances that you have at the present, those that you are not yet able to change. Perhaps the Serenity Prayer sums it up best:

> God grant me the serenity to accept the things I cannot change;
> Courage to change the things I can; and wisdom to know the
>   difference.
> Living one day at a time;
> Enjoying one moment at a time;
> Accepting hardships as the pathway to peace;
> Taking, as He did, this sinful world as it is, not as I would have it;

Trusting that He will make all things right if I surrender to His Will;
That I may be reasonably happy in this life and supremely happy
  with Him
Forever in the next. Amen (Niebuhr 1943).

Be good to yourself. Give yourself the same level of nurturing that you would give your spouse, child, pet, or best friend. Fill your mind with self-supporting thoughts. The way you view yourself matters most because you are the one person guaranteed to be with you for the rest of your life. Your belief in yourself and your abilities will give you the greatest chance for success in overcoming adversity.

Understand and accept your limitations, and insist that those who share your life do the same. If you have a chronic condition that causes fatigue, sleep deprivation is not an option for you. If you try to push yourself to live up to your own unrealistic expectations or those of others, you will eventually pay the price. Make sure those around you understand the limitations that you have. Don't try to put on a brave front. Be honest about the realities of your condition, with others, and with yourself.

The "Spoon Theory"

One tool that can provide others with insight into your illness or injury is the spoon theory. Christine Miserandino, a lupus patient, created it as a way to describe her daily life to a friend. She made her point by giving the friend 12 spoons, the allotment for the day. Healthy people have an unlimited supply of spoons, but those dealing with a chronic illness have a limited number. Miserandino asked her friend to imagine having lupus and then took away a spoon for each activity of the day, such as making breakfast or taking a shower. Half of the spoons were gone before her friend even made it to work (Miserandino 2003). As you can see, you must select the spoons you want to give up carefully and pace yourself throughout the day.

It is your responsibility to educate those around you, especially your loved ones. Patience is key. You may get frustrated when others can't relate to your challenges, but keep in mind that they cannot feel what you feel. If your symptoms are invisible, you have a different set of difficulties, and you have undoubtedly done a lot of tongue-biting. You may look fine on the outside while experiencing excruciating pain, cognitive impairment, fatigue, dizziness, or other symptoms hidden on the inside.

When others cannot feel your symptoms and cannot see evidence of your suffering, it is less real to them. Some may go as far as to dismiss your complaints or doubt that anything is wrong. Although this kind of treatment is hurtful, you have an opportunity to enlighten those who need it. To learn more about coping with invisible disabilities, visit www.butyoudontlooksick .com or www.InvisibleDisabilities.org. Stacy Taylor, MSW, LCSW, and Robert Epstein, PhD, explore this topic in their book *Living Well with a Hidden Disability: Transcending Doubt and Shame and Reclaiming Your Life.*

Try to make your condition as real and as quantifiable as possible. Be as specific as possible with the information you provide. When all else fails, try to find the humor in those who are not enlightened. When I asked Milton to describe some of the less-than-insightful questions and observations he has heard, we had a good laugh. His favorites range from, "Does it hurt?" to "That's what you get for being part of a motorcycle gang."

The Role of Humor

Not only is humor a great coping mechanism, but laughter provides physiological benefits. It releases endorphins into the brain and gives the cardiovascular system a good workout. It also distracts us from whatever is troubling us. Norman Cousins talks about the physiology of laughter in his book *Anatomy of an Illness as Perceived by the Patient.* The Bible addresses the healing effects of joy in Proverbs 17:22: "A merry heart does good, like medicine, but a broken spirit dries the bones."

You have the power to fill your life with laughter. You can choose to surround yourself with people who make you laugh and to avoid those who bring you down. You also have choices in selecting television programs and movies. Lighthearted sitcoms and movies are much better choices than dark dramas or news programs when you are seeking a reprieve from your symptoms. You can lose yourself in laughter and feel better physically before you even realize what has happened.

15 Strategies for Coping with Debilitating Symptoms

1. Let go and let God. When you are in the depths of despair, remember that you are never alone. Surrender your troubles to God and ask Him to help you carry your burden.

2. Don't let your illness or injury define you. Think of all of your attributes that have nothing to do with your disability—the traits and skills that you have accumulated throughout your life. Nobody and nothing can take those away from you.

3. Instead of focusing on what has been taken away from you, focus on what you have and make the most of it. Don't look at whether the glass is half full or half empty. Reinvest in yourself, and fill that glass.

4. Build a healthy support system. Surround yourself with people who believe in you. Remove toxic people from your life. Find others who have similar symptoms through local support groups and online support groups or forums. They know what you are going through.

5. Include a pet in your support system. Pets provide unconditional love, and they don't judge their humans. Be sure to select a pet that fits into your lifestyle for your sake and the pet's sake. A great way to do this is by visiting a shelter with different kinds of pets. Spend time with several cats or dogs to make sure that you and your new fur baby are well suited for each other. You can search for shelters and for specific pets and breeds at www.petfinder.com.

6. Educate yourself as much as possible about your condition. When you arm yourself with information, you feel more secure and in control of your life. You are also in a better position to offer insight to others.

7. Consult a therapist, counselor, or member of the clergy. The people closest to you do not have the objectivity of a professional. They may be affected by your condition to the extent that they do not have enough left in them to listen objectively. You can vent to a professional safely and confidentially and without worrying that you are burdening him with your problems.

8. If you do not have the resources to seek professional help, you may benefit from a Stephen Minister. The Stephen Ministry program is a nationwide, nondenominational outreach network that trains laypersons to provide Christ-centered care to people who are experiencing difficulties. Many large churches have a Stephen Ministry program that is open to everyone in the community. Stephen Ministers receive fifty hours of training on topics such as grief, illness, loss of employment, childbirth, loneliness, anxiety, and depression. Trained Stephen Ministers serve under the supervision of Stephen leaders and other Stephen Ministers, and they keep all information confidential.

9. Don't depend on others for happiness. True happiness has to come from within. Happiness is your personal journey and responsibility. To some degree, you have to depend on others for physical and emotional support, though. Seek support from a network of people so that no single person becomes overwhelmed.

10. Don't look for reasons or blame. Don't waste time and energy looking for reasons that explain why you are suffering, unless the answers provide the key to your healing. In most cases, there are no answers. Don't allow others to blame you for your condition or to ask what you did to bring it upon yourself.

11. Don't apologize for your condition. You have no reason to apologize—you are not any more to blame than anyone else. This is easier said than done if you fear that you may be inconveniencing others. But unless you are intentionally inconveniencing others, it is not your fault.

12. If your condition is undiagnosed, don't minimize it to yourself or to anyone else. During my long period of misdiagnosis and no diagnosis, I was ashamed and filled with self-loathing. I didn't feel that I had the right to experience those symptoms and inconvenience other people without a valid diagnosis. Don't do this to yourself. Your symptoms and suffering are just as real as those of people who have been diagnosed.

13. *Do your best to maintain a positive attitude and to visualize healing.* The mind-body connection is stronger than we realize. Your unconscious mind is working behind the scenes, sending cognitive messages that reverberate throughout the body. Use your emotions to facilitate healing.

14. *Use relaxation techniques to put your body in a healing state.* Listen to soothing music; try meditation or deep muscle relaxation. For more information on relaxation techniques, visit healthylifestyle.upmc.com/ Stress Relaxation.htm. Additional relaxation tools are listed in the Resources at a Glance section.

15. *Write your thoughts, hopes, fears, and dreams in a journal.* Like relaxation techniques, journaling allows you to release negative emotions. Anxiety and anger are disruptive to sleep, something you cannot do without. Journaling gives you the freedom to say whatever is on your mind without concern for others' reactions.

Managing Pain

Pain management is an important part of coping with a medical condition. Pain is not always curable, but it can be managed. Pain generally has two origins, nociceptive and neuropathic. Nociceptive pain occurs when the body's nervous system is working properly and tells the brain that there is an injury to the body such as a laceration, blunt force trauma, or back injury like a disk herniation or a pulled sacroiliac joint. Neuropathic pain is caused by abnormal nerve activity. The body tells the brain that pain is present although the source cannot be identified. Neuropathic pain conditions include reflex sympathetic dystrophy, fibromyalgia, and interstitial cystitis (Helm 2009). In rare cases, pain has a psychological origin such as depression, or it is caused by a psychiatric condition such as a somatoform disorder or hypochondriasis.

Treatment for pain varies widely and should be customized for the kind of pain the patient is experiencing. Pain management regimens fall into three categories: noninvasive, nondrug treatments; noninvasive pharmaceutical therapies; and invasive techniques.

Pain-Management Regimens

Noninvasive, nondrug treatments

Exercise provides natural pain relief by releasing endorphins in the brain that flood the body. It specifically helps with joint pain by building muscles around and lubricating the joints.

Physical therapy rehabilitates painful joints and muscles and relieves pain slowly over time.

Ergonomic intervention eliminates pain by getting to the source of repetitive-motion or heavy-lifting injuries.

Manual techniques such as massage therapy, chiropractic treatments, and osteopathy use physical touch to treat deep-muscle tissue pain.

Behavioral modification recognizes the strong mind-body connection and includes cognitive therapy, hypnotherapy, biofeedback, and other relaxation techniques to optimize the patient's physical and emotional response to pain. To find a certified hypnotherapist, visit http://www.asch.net. You can search for a certified professional by area of expertise, including pain management.

Cutaneous stimulation is superficial treatment to the skin, usually involving heat or cold packs. This method is often combined with manual techniques or exercise.

Electrotherapy is the use of electrical currents to speed healing and ease pain. The most common form of electrotherapy is transcutaneous electrical nerve stimulation (TENS). This technique targets the sensory nervous system with low-voltage electrical stimulation.

Acupuncture is most commonly used to treat musculoskeletal pain and headaches. This method requires the insertion of thin needles into the skin at designated points called meridians, which correspond to certain organs and areas of the body. Acupuncture has been used for centuries to diagnose and treat diseases and to restore balance to the body.

Noninvasive pharmaceutical pain relief

Nonnarcotic analgesics include acetaminophen and nonsteroidal anti-inflammatory drugs (NSAIDs), and many are available without a prescription. Long-term use can result in kidney damage. Check with your doctor before taking over-the-counter medication.

Muscle relaxants are used to calm muscle spasms and usually cause drowsiness, making them more appropriate for short-term use.

Oral steroids such as Prednisone are sometimes used for pain management because of their anti-inflammatory benefits, usually in an autoimmune disease such as arthritis. Oral steroids are not intended as long-term therapy because of their side effects. A short-term dose, called a burst pack, offers quick relief while minimizing side effects.

Narcotics are used primarily for acute or postoperative pain because of their sedating effect and the risk of addiction.

Antidepressants and anticonvulsants are effective treatments for neuropathic pain. Tricyclic antidepressants were the preferred therapy until SSRIs (selective serotonin reuptake inhibitors) were introduced, offering fewer side effects. Lyrica is perhaps the most popular drug in this category. It is targeted to treat nerve pain but also helps manage seizures. It has side effects, but the drowsiness gets better after the body has time to adjust, usually within several days.

Invasive treatments

Injections deliver drugs such as steroids and anesthetics directly to the nerve, joint, or epidural area. They are used as diagnostic tools and for short-term pain relief.

Surgically implanted electrotherapy devices offer the pain relief of a TENS unit internally.

Implantable opioid infusion pumps deliver pain relief directly to the affected nerve. Because of the powerful narcotics involved, this treatment is a last resort.

Radiofrequency ablation uses electrical currents to heat nerve tissue in an effort to minimize the pain signals coming from that area.

Surgery is considered after all other options have been exhausted, but in some cases it is necessary, as in joint replacement (Cutler 2006).

For information on treatments by condition

Visit www.nationalpainfoundation.org and click on My Treatment, then select a pain category. This site offers detailed treatment information for each category and provides a tool to search particular conditions. The site also has a search tool to find pain management specialists by location.

If you are suffering from chronic pain, you have a number of options, but you should weigh them carefully. The lowest-risk, least-invasive treatments should be exhausted first. However, you must consider the benefit-to-risk ratio and educate yourself as much as possible when selecting your treatment. If there is a reputable pain management treatment center in your community, your PCP can make a referral. A good pain management facility will use a team approach and integrate as many low-risk, noninvasive techniques as possible. Be wary of any facility or practitioner who wants to keep you on narcotics without adjunct therapy. The ideal multidisciplinary pain management center team will include...

- a physician with expertise in pain management (neurologist, anesthesiologist, or psychiatrist)

- a registered nurse

- a psychologist with expertise in family counseling

- physical and occupational therapists
- a biofeedback therapist
- a massage therapist

Services provided by the pain-management center should include the following:

- regional anesthesia and oral medications as needed, but not without adjunct therapy
- physical and occupational therapy
- counseling, including family and group counseling
- TENS therapy
- biofeedback treatment
- massage therapy
- relaxation training and stress management
- education and aftercare (Managing 2009)

Managing the Effect of Disabilty on Marriage and Family

The American Chronic Pain Association places great emphasis on family counseling as part of pain management treatment. Chronic pain, or any debilitating condition for that matter, can wreak havoc on interpersonal relationships. The loss experienced by the patient reverberates and affects everyone in her life. Family dynamics change when an illness or an injury upsets the balance. Family counseling is very important, especially when children are involved. It's scary enough for adults to deal with a disability, but children are completely at the mercy of the adults around them. They see their family's lives in a state of upheaval but are powerless to do anything about it. They need a safe place where they can share their feelings openly without guilt or concern.

Seventy-five percent of marriages affected by chronic illness end in divorce (Prater 2008). Disability is overwhelming to a marriage, unless that disability is present before the marriage. The problem arises when both the husband and wife are healthy for a number of years and become accustomed to that life. And then suddenly, disaster strikes, and life as the happily married couple has known it is over.

The healthy spouse is frustrated and thinks, *This isn't what I bargained for.* The healthy spouse suddenly has more responsibility while also grieving the loss of the once-healthy partner. The disabled spouse, who already feels devalued by her condition, feels even more diminished by her spouse's frustration. Both are angry but cannot get mad at something inanimate like illness, so they project their anger onto one another. Anger and resentment build until the disability overshadows the marriage.

Undiagnosed or misdiagnosed conditions present a daunting challenge to families. This factor contributed to the demise of my own marriage, because Joe and I saw no finite end to the situation. We had nowhere to direct our frustrations because for years we didn't know what we were dealing with. The ambiguity of the undiagnosed condition felt like a moving target for both of us.

Add to the mix the different ways men and women express their emotions, and you have a recipe for disaster. Men find it harder to communicate and are more likely to become isolated. They have difficulty expressing delicate emotions and often show anger when they are feeling concern. Women take the anger personally. They internalize and try to take responsibility for their husbands' emotions and feel they have done something wrong. Communication continues to erode as both just try to get through each day. Finally, there is nothing left.

The 25 percent of marriages that survive a disability have a strong foundation. A marriage is like a house—if it has a strong foundation, it can withstand anything. Some marriages even thrive in the face of adversity as each spouse develops more respect and admiration for the other while they fight the battle together. Families can grow closer as parents watch their children grow into strong, compassionate adults.

You can strengthen your foundation and your family's bond by helping your loved ones help you.

- *Ask for help.* Be very specific when telling loved ones what you need. Don't assume that others will know what you need because they love you.

- *Realize your loved ones are hurting and grieving too.* They have experienced a loss, a change in dynamics. Don't take their grief personally, and don't feel guilty because you cannot do the things you did before your illness or injury. Allow loved ones to be angry at the situation.

- *Build the largest support system you can.* You need to seek help from as many sources as possible. You cannot accept help from just one person—this is a recipe for caregiver burnout. Try to create a rotating schedule for assistance from loved ones.

- *Whenever possible, seek emotional support from someone who does not live in your household.* Those who are closest to you and most affected by your condition cannot be the most objective. They are too close to the situation and are often overwhelmed by additional responsibility. When you need to vent, try to do so with a friend, a member of the clergy, or a mental-health professional…someone who is more removed from your situation.

- *Try to offset the additional responsibility your loved ones now have.* Look at what you can do to keep a balance in household responsibilities. For example, if you have mobility issues and your spouse must take on more housework, perhaps you can assume responsibility for paying bills and creating grocery lists.

- *Encourage your loved ones to take breaks from the responsibility.* Give them time away from the situation to recharge their batteries. An afternoon of leisure time with no responsibility can work wonders for a stressed-out caregiver.

- *Seek help together.* Family counseling can be very helpful when dealing with a debilitating illness or injury. If counseling is not an option or seems intimidating, consider a support group for your condition—and attend meetings as a family or as a couple. Support-group meetings can be very validating for the entire family, because other support-group members can empathize with the entire situation.

Life does not have to stop for an illness or injury. It might slow down or veer off into an entirely different direction. That new direction may provide rewards and blessing you could never have imagined. Don't be afraid of change, of embracing the new you. You can have a good life if you make the conscious decision to do so—and if you find happiness wherever you can.

Chapter 10

Understanding God's Will

Finding Meaning in Your Experience

After Dr. Watkins began treating my autonomic disorder in early 2002, I noticed small but significant strides. Several weeks after I began the Zoloft-Florinef regimen, I became slightly more tolerant of stimuli and could go into small stores for short periods of time. I still had to walk with a cane because of the spinning and swimming sensations. The cane helped me feel more connected to the ground and more inside my body.

I began to enjoy Pilates classes more because I did not get as disoriented. The exercise didn't cause the disorientation—the stimuli did, although they were minimal in the small studio with its dim lighting. I must have looked really strange walking with a cane into the studio after Linda dropped me off and then proceeding to take the advanced mat class. My muscular strength was very good from all of the power yoga and Pilates, but I constantly felt as if everything was spinning and swimming.

Every couple of months, I noticed slight improvement. I could do something that had not been possible before: eating in a small restaurant, walking halfway down the street without becoming disoriented by the passing scenery, shopping in a drugstore. Even with improved functioning, I was still very guarded, though. I was afraid to get my hopes up for fear that I would lose the progress or that the medication would stop working. I was afraid to trust that my good fortune was real. As always, Linda was attuned to what I could and could not handle physically. She could look at a store or restaurant and know whether or not I could manage it just by observing the stimuli, particularly the noise level and lighting. For example, my chances were better with natural lighting than fluorescent lighting.

I couldn't walk into a grocery store and select my own food for about four years. When I finally triumphed and completed a grocery-shopping excursion with Linda and Mitchell, I was ecstatic. Linda, watching with fascination, said, "I will never complain about going to the grocery store ever again. I now realize it is a privilege."

As my progress continued, I was able to tolerate larger stores and restaurants with a cane, and smaller stores without one. I even improved enough to go into small places by myself, without anybody helping me navigate. Linda could stay in the car with Mitchell while I went into the post office or a convenience store. This was in sharp contrast to the arrangement we'd had when my functioning level was at its lowest, when Linda had to go into most places for me.

With the improvement, I was much more comfortable when Joe and I went to church, and no longer had to sit at the very end of the back pew in case I had to step out. At my lowest point, I had struggled to stay in the sanctuary because of the stimuli. When it became too much, I slipped out the back and sat in a small room until the service was over. (Ours was a very small church with a very small sanctuary.) When my symptoms were at their worst, the pastor looked very far away, but as the Zoloft and Florinef worked their magic, he appeared closer, my vision was less blurry, and I improved enough to handle both Sunday school and church. Eventually, I stopped using my cane at church, to the joy of fellow parishioners. Joe and I were able to attend more church functions, and I even played the clarinet during some of the services and other events. Life was definitely getting better.

As the months progressed, I was able to walk much farther. Instead of getting disoriented walking to the end of the driveway, I enjoyed continuous milestones with walking around the neighborhood. Eventually, I could walk one mile, then two. Life was getting better all the time, and my newfound independence removed pressure from both Joe and me.

By late 2003, I was frustrated because I could walk much farther than

I could drive. My 15-year-old car had only 47,000 miles on it because of all the years I'd been unable to drive. I sometimes started the car and drove it a couple of houses down the street just to keep it in running condition, but I hadn't tried to drive anywhere I wanted to go. Finally, I decided to give it a try and was delighted to find that I could go one mile safely if I stayed at 25 mph. That first short trip was liberating, exhilarating, and terrifying all at the same time. I tried driving every few days to gauge my improvement, but it was very slow going. Four months later, I could drive two miles, then three miles, and by mid-2004, I could drive four miles.

After my marriage ended in mid-2004, I moved to a more central neighborhood, where everything I could possibly need is within four miles. As a matter of fact, just about everything I could possibly need is within two miles: doctors, hospitals, grocery stores, drugstores, restaurants, the veterinary emergency clinic, a neighborhood park, swimming pools, a nice shopping mall, and several shopping centers.

Just before I moved, Mitchell started school and Linda went back to work full-time. Somehow, I had known for years that the timing would work out this way. By the time Linda was no longer available as my driver, I was almost independent. During the two-week gap when I needed a driver, Linda's friend, who was between jobs, stepped in. It all worked out perfectly.

In my new home, with everything so convenient, I was like a kid in a candy store! I drove everywhere I could possibly drive and ran countless errands. I'll never forget driving to the grocery store for the first time, walking in all by myself with nobody helping me navigate, selecting my own groceries, and driving home, all without assistance. Incredible! And I was beside myself with joy when I drove to the massive Target shopping center four miles away. It is so huge that in December, I can start at one end and have my Christmas shopping completed by the time I reach the other end. I was in a state of shopaholic bliss!

I thoroughly enjoyed excursions to Lowe's and Home Depot while I was discovering the joys of lawn care. I found that I got more pleasure from buying lawn tools than clothing. How did that happen? My biggest shopping triumph was a trip to Sam's Club several weeks after I moved.

Sam's had always presented a sensory challenge because of its lighting and sheer size, but I had improved so much that I could finally shop there unassisted and not have to leave because of the disorienting stimuli. During that first visit, I perused every aisle, not wanting to miss anything. By the time I finished, tears of joy were streaming down my face.

New and Old Friends

By late 2004, I was ready to find a new companion, a new fur baby to love. I knew I wanted another German shepherd, so I visited the German Shepherd Rescue of Central Alabama (GSRCA) after passing a rigorous home inspection. When I met the second group of dogs, there he was—the most beautiful golden teddy bear I had ever seen. It was love at first sight!

I found out later that this magnificent creature had been one hour away from euthanasia when GSRCA rescued him. Beau and I adopted each other a month after his rescue. On the way home from GSRCA, I called friends and family and announced, "It's a boy!"

Five years later, Beau and I are still living happily ever after. He offers boundless, unconditional love and affection and asks for very little in return. He loves people and car rides. We are a canine—human match made in heaven!

Linda is happily remarried, to her high-school sweetheart, Wes. Mitchell is a joyful 11-year-old, straight-A student with plans to attend Harvard Business School. They live two hours away, and I really miss them, but we keep in touch via phone, text, and e-mails and get together whenever we can.

The Zoloft and Florinef regimen has gradually continued working its magic. I have regained most of my life, and I can drive for as long as an hour and at speeds up to 60 mph. I still have trouble on large highways with several lanes because everything is so open and because of the multiple lines on the road. I need narrower roads with buildings and trees along the side to break up the visual overload of the open space. I can attend events in crowded, noisy places, and I can eat in noisy restaurants. I can shop at the mall at Christmastime, and I can shop in Wal-Mart during busy weekend hours. And I can shop in the grocery store two hours before kickoff time for the annual Alabama-Auburn football game. Even without an autonomic disorder, many people cannot do that!

I still have a little bit of trouble in crowded airports and a lot of trouble with the dehydration associated with air travel. People with autonomic disorders have only about 80 percent of the body fluids that others have. Dehydration hits autonomic patients much harder and is much more difficult to overcome. Dr. Coghlan noted in my tilt-table test report in 2001 that "this patient must not get dehydrated." Over the years, whenever an ulcerative colitis flare-up caused dehydration and the associated symptoms of low blood pressure, lightheadedness, and headache, I went to an urgent-care clinic and got IV fluids and usually felt better within a few days. But I experienced a significant health setback from December 2007 to June 2008, triggered by a severe dehydration episode that was followed by an even more dehydrating plane trip. This setback took months to overcome, and I continue to take precautions to avoid dehydration at all costs.

Finding Meaning in the Journey

Overall, life is amazing. I have most of my life back after losing it for nine long years. During that time, I didn't really have a life; it was more of an existence. Although Dr. Watkins diagnosed my symptoms after seven years, the treatment worked very gradually. I did not begin to live a reasonably normal life until I had been on the medication for about two years. I can't begin to describe how rewarding life is the second time around! I appreciate everything so much more. I will never again take for granted privileges such as staying in the sanctuary during a church service, driving a car, shopping in a store, walking through the neighborhood, and sitting in a room with fluorescent lighting.

To the surprise of others, I never wondered why I was losing years of my life while I was experiencing the symptoms. I just wanted to focus on getting better and not waste time on a question that had no answer. I didn't question God's will, although I prayed a lot for healing. I prayed and prayed for a quick fix that never happened, but I began to see results when I prayed for direction.

Once I regained my life, I became much more introspective and wanted to find meaning in my journey. Why did God give me this experience? Was it because He knew I was strong enough, or did I become strong enough because of the journey? Did He actually give me the experience and the gift of overcoming my disability? How much of my recovery was due to His mercy? How much could be attributed to wonderful doctors like Dr. Wyatt, Dr. Watkins, and Dr. Pappas, or to Dr. Coghlan's evaluation of my tilt-table test? How much was due to my own tenacity? What did God expect me to learn from my journey? What did He expect me to do with this experience? The more my health improved, the more I felt that I needed to do something with my gift. It was almost as if I needed to pay back my good fortune or, better yet, pay it forward. I had mulled over the idea of writing a book but had never seriously pursued it.

One day during my self-discovery phase, I was reading Joyce Meyer's book *Approval Addiction*. In a section entitled "God is Looking for Experienced Help," Meyer writes, "When we go to work for God in His kingdom, He will use everything in our past, no matter how painful it was. He considers it experience. We have gone through some difficult things, and those things qualify us to help take someone else through them too" (237). When I read that powerful passage, I could almost feel God kicking my complacent backside and telling me to hurry up and write the book. In that instant, I knew what I needed to do. But I had no idea how to get started.

Once again, I prayed very hard for direction. About three weeks later, I mentioned my desire to a fellow parishioner, who suggested that I talk to her co-worker and local author, Austin Boyd. A week later, the three of us had lunch, and Austin gave me a "New Writer's 101" mini-course. He provided the mentoring I desperately needed, and I have never looked back.

Within a few months, I attended the Mount Hermon Christian Writer's Conference with 450 other writers. I quickly realized the extent of my physical progress; all 450 of us attended evening sessions together in a large auditorium, and we ate meals together in a large dining hall. Talk about sensory overload! But I got along just fine. I knew without a doubt that I had regained my life. And because of the contacts I made during the conference, I found an agent and publisher. Everything fell into place so neatly that it was almost eerie. It didn't take a rocket scientist to figure out God's plan for me. (By the way, Austin is a rocket scientist!)

Experiencing God's Plan

Ivy Larson is very clear on God's plan for her. When she brought her multiple sclerosis into remission with a healthy diet, she felt called to help others. She believes that her MS and recovery happened for a reason, and she is grateful for the sense of purpose that they have provided. Ivy recognizes that she would not be the person she is today without having faced adversity and come out on the other side. She believes that when faced with a challenge, the way you deal with that challenge is what shapes you as a person. She is inspired by people who have faced challenges far greater than hers and come out stronger, better people.

Ivy found a hidden blessing during her painful journey. Her mother had always been a very spiritual and religious person, but her father wasn't nearly so religious. But when Ivy was diagnosed with MS, her father called upon everyone he knew and asked them to pray for her. He became very spiritual after Ivy's diagnosis and then became an even bigger believer in God after he saw the positive effect that her diagnosis and healing diet had on others. Today, his faith is very strong.

Karen Grove has also followed God's command after improving from a 5 percent functioning level to 100 percent after a grueling battle with fibromyalgia. Her improvement was the result of the natural regimen she created, the Grove Approach. As Karen found more and more healing tools, including yoga, massage, and nutrition, she was able to build an entire fibromyalgia healing program. She credits God with guiding her every step of the way and placing the right resources in her path. She believes her suffering was an important and necessary part of His plan for her; it was the catalyst for her natural treatment for fibromyalgia. She was backed into a corner and forced to find relief when no physician could figure out a way to help her and is now grateful for all that she has learned, but she continues to learn from others.

Steve Marshburn, president of LS&ESSI, says there is no doubt in his mind that his injury was part of God's plan for him. Forty years ago, he was struck by lightning while inside a building on a sunny day, not during storm season, and with the storm at least ten miles away. Lightning injuries are rare enough, but this one completely defied scientific reasoning. Steve's injury resulted in seizures, cognitive deficits, cancer, and horrendous pain throughout his body, including frequent migraines.

Instead of focusing on his own distress, Steve wondered how many others were suffering with similar symptoms and no doctor who could help because of the rarity of lightning injuries. He founded a support group 20 years ago that exploded into a worldwide network after he appeared on the *Today Show*. Lightning Strike and Electric Shock Survivors, International (LS&ESSI) is a nonprofit organization, now with 1575 members worldwide.

In 2000, Steve began taking a new anticonvulsant that stopped his seizures the same day, and he has not had another seizure since that time. Six years later, one of his physicians asked him how long it had been since he had driven a car, and Steve responded, "Nineteen very long years." The physician determined that Steve could drive safely and authorized him to get his license back. That was one of the happiest moments of Steve's life. He felt, and still feels, that he got his manhood back when he could drive again. And of course, he savors that privilege even more because it is so much sweeter the second time around. Steve feels truly blessed by all of the good things in his life and believes he has been rewarded several times over for his hard work as president and founder of LS&ESSI. He brags about his global family of lightning and electric shock survivors.

Milton Anthony believes his nearly fatal bombing was a wake-up call from God. Before the bombing, Milton lived on the edge as a "national enforcer" of an international motorcycle club. He had dropped out of high school to spend all of his time hanging out with his club brothers and battling rival clubs. He thought this was how he wanted to live and thrived on the feelings of machismo and invincibility, not to mention his sense of belonging. He enjoyed this life despite the four attempts that had been made on his life.

But the fifth attempt changed everything, as told in the previous chapter. Because he had come so close to death, Milton could only surmise that God must have spared his life for a reason and had a mission for him. His search for his life's purpose led him to complete his GED and his bachelor's and master's degrees and to become a licensed counselor. He has dedicated his life to helping others and provides counseling and pain-management training. Today, Milton is at peace, finally understanding God's plan for him.

Ruth Kriz explains her journey with the rhetorical question: "Why waste perfectly good suffering?" Ruth endured 11 years of what is commonly known as interstitial cystitis (IC). Her symptoms were nearly unbearable; she could not wear anything tight around her waist for years. When traditional treatment failed to alleviate her symptoms, she delved more deeply into her mysterious condition.

She started networking with two microbiologists. They have come to believe that the underlying cause of the chronic bladder disorder is actually a bartonella-like co-infection of Lyme disease. They developed a protocol for treating it, using antibiotics and nutritional supplements to repair the damaged bladder wall and boost the immune system. Today, Ruth is symptom-free and successfully treating others who have this painful and often debilitating condition. Although Ruth would not want to relive those difficult 11 years, she says, "I am who I am because of my experience." She points out that Jesus was moved by compassion and that we should live by His example.

Ivy, Karen, Steve, Milton, and Ruth serve God by using their painful experiences to help others. And this, in turn, brings them additional blessings. As Steve says, "When I am assisting others, I forget about my own pain." Rick Warren challenges all of us to become God's instruments in his book *The Purpose-Driven Life*, and refers to 2 Corinthians 1:4: "He comforts us in all our troubles, so that we can comfort those in any trouble with the comfort we ourselves have received from God."

Warren points out that our most painful experiences are the ones God wants us to use to help others (Warren, 247).

The "Why" of Suffering

Does God give us our painful experiences, or are they created by man? When I asked Laurie Todd about her difficult, simultaneous battles with cancer and her insurer, her response was more pragmatic. She does not believe that God gave her cancer as a test, punishment, or learning experience. Laurie describes cancer as "the organism's response to a lifetime bombardment of chemicals." She does not believe that God chose her for this journey, but that she is the best person for the job. As a result of Laurie's successful appeal for out-of-network insurance coverage, she now wins appeals for others who face battles with their insurance providers.

One of my mother's friends offered a similar explanation for Mom's cancer, telling her, "God did not do this to you. Cancer is man-made." That simple statement offered Mom and our entire family a great deal of comfort. We could not fathom the possibility the God had given Mom cancer. She was the most selfless person we had ever known. She did not deserve the suffering she had to endure—not that anybody deserves it. Dad, my brothers, and I continually asked, "Why her?" Of all the people on earth, why did this have to happen to someone so sweet and caring, so good to the core?

Lawrence W. Wilson ponders this in his book *Why Me? Straight Talk about Suffering.* He reminds us that suffering is inevitable; there is no escape. My Stephen Ministry training class agrees. During one session, we concluded that there is no way around physical and emotional pain. We can't go around it or under it; we have to go through it. We cannot expect to go through life without a number of trials. The longer we are alive, the more adversity we have to face.

My father recently lamented that my older brother and I had been through a lot during the last two years. My response? "At our stage in life, who hasn't?" By midlife, most of us have experienced loss of a loved one, illness, divorce, loss of employment, or any combination of these events. Recognizing that adversity is a part of life may not take the sting out of our pain, but it just may give us the strength to get through it, knowing that better days are ahead. Life is a series of ups and downs, a combination of pain and pleasure.

In *Why Me?* Wilson explores the analogous parent–child and God–His children relationships. He wonders what would happen if God's behavior fit snugly within the confines of our understanding. What would happen to us if God acted only according to the will of His creatures? Probably the same thing that happens when parents act according to the will of their children. Wilson reminds us that God knows more than we do, and we cannot compare our minds to His (Wilson, 50).

In *Direction: Discernment for the Decisions of Your Life* Cheri Cowell reminds us that we could not love God unconditionally if He gave us everything we wanted. We would be like spoiled children if everything were easy and required no effort. We must have faith in His wisdom, even when we don't understand it. God's grace gives us peeks into His wisdom and His will, but we will not see the grand masterpiece until we get to heaven. In the meantime, we can pray for insight into His wisdom and tell Him what we don't understand and ask for clarity. We can also allow others to help us see what we cannot see when we are too close to the situation.

God does not cause our suffering. In fact, He never intended for us to suffer when He created the earth in perfect harmony and asked us to live in the way that He created. But when we breached that contract we usurped His authority, leaving Him with no choice but to allow suffering (Cowell 2007). Does this mean that God is forsaking us? Not at all. God is working within us to give us strength when we are facing adversity. When Satan tormented Paul with a thorn in his side, Paul pleaded for God to remove the thorn three times. In 2 Corinthians 12:9, God told him, "My grace is sufficient for you, for My strength is made perfect in weakness."

Knowing God Better

We can gain power by relying more fully on God. My friend Phyllis has lost two husbands to cancer. She and Carey were married for only two months when he was diagnosed with terminal colon cancer. He fought with everything he had but passed away two years later. During his final days, Carey talked to the angels and told Phyllis, "Jesus is coming to get me. Will you be okay?" Carey was not afraid to die; he was ready to be with the Lord. As Carey took his last breath, Phyllis saw a white dove outside looking in the window at Carey. She saw this as a sign that Carey was going to be okay because white doves are so uncommon in Alabama.

After Carey passed away and Phyllis had begun to heal, she found love again. She and Don were married for eight blissful years before he was diagnosed with glioblastoma multiforme, a deadly brain cancer. Don also lived for two years after his diagnosis, but they were hard years. The cancer affected his cognition, motor skills, and personality. When I asked Phyllis how her experiences had affected her relationship with God, she responded, "They strengthened my relationship with God." She now more than ever believes in the hereafter and feels the grace of the Holy Spirit with her. She also believes that Carey and Don are spending time together, telling tales and having fun.

How can we live according to God's will when we are hurting physically or emotionally and just don't understand why we have to bear this burden? Knowing God's will is about knowing God. If we want to know God's will, we need to focus more on knowing God than on knowing His will. As we get to know God better, His will begins to reveal itself. In Colossians 1:3-14, Paul shows us how this spiraling process works and directs us toward five points in the "spiral," as follows.

The "Five R's": Knowing God and Understanding His Will

1. We *remember* God's goodness and the way He has touched our lives or the lives of others. When we are blinded by crisis, we may need to look at our past blessings or seek encouragement from the experience of others. Support groups provide a great forum for remembering and witnessing God's goodness. Inspirational stories, such as those of Ivy, Karen, Ruth, Milton, and Steve help us remember God's grace

2. We *realize* that we are in a state of growth. Whatever is going on around us is bigger than us and our situation. It is not about us and what

we are doing, but what God is doing in our lives to help us grow. In His wisdom, He sees our need for growth. When we reach this realization, we become more humble and open to opportunities for growth. We become aware of God's larger purpose for us with others.

3. We *release* control of the situation and turn it over to God, as Jesus did in the Garden of Gethsemane. In Luke 22:42 He says, "Take this cup away from Me: nevertheless not My will, but Yours, be done." Although we may never have the level of trust that Jesus had, we must strive to trust God's will, even when we do not understand it during a time of crisis. God does not always answer our prayers the way we would like for Him to do so, or in a way that we understand. His wisdom may become apparent years later, as in my case. For years, I could not understand why He would not help me find a diagnosis and cure. But now I understand perfectly—my medical journey was at the core of His plan for me.

4. We *review* our behavior to ensure that it pleases God and honors Him. Colossians 1:10-14 advises us to live a life worthy of and pleasing to God, bearing fruit in every good work, and growing in the knowledge of God. This is a tall order when we are hurting and struggling to get through each day. We may become angry at God when we believe He is forsaking us. If you find yourself in this position, step outside of your troubles to help others. There is truth to the saying, "The best way to forget about your own adversity is by helping others." You will most likely feel better about your own situation due to increased perspective and the feeling of accomplishment, of making a difference. This is God's will at work.

5. We *rest* and see God's hand in our lives. We take time to reflect on God's goodness and what He has done for us. Our busy lives are not conducive to this very important step. Once the crisis has passed, we are ready to get back to life as usual. But how can we appreciate our blessings if we don't slow down and give thanks? I am guilty of this lack of reflection and introspection. I am so busy making up

for lost time that I fail to stop and think of how blessed I am to have my life back. But sometimes, while shopping in a large store or driving on a highway, I marvel at how far I've come and I give thanks for God's goodness.

Each of us has our own experience of living according to God's will. Our interpretations are shaped by our experience. My interpretation would be very different had it not been for my medical odyssey. Prior to it, I had no idea what God intended for me to do with my time on earth. Like many people, I was just going through life without much thought to its meaning.

My medical journey changed all that, and now I seek meaning for my life and its purpose. Instead of muddling through life, I am now on a mission—a mission to help others avoid some of the pitfalls I encountered during my search for the correct diagnosis and treatment. I aspire to be like Ivy, Karen, Steve, Milton, and Ruth…who now serve God by helping others with the lessons they learned while overcoming the adversities they experienced. In some small way, I hope this book allows me to follow their examples and to live according to God's will. And I hope it will do the same for you.

Resources at a Glance

—

Helpful Charts
for Recordkeeping

—

Acknowledgments

—

Guide to Medical
Terminology in This Book

—

References

—

Index

Resources at a Glance

General Health

www.nlm.nih.gov (National Library of Medicine)

www.partnershipforhealthcare.org/resources/factsheets.asp (Partnership for Healthcare Excellence)

Misdiagnosis and Practitioners

How Doctors Think by Jerome Groopman

The Intelligent Patient's Guide to the Doctor-Patient Relationship: Learning How to Talk So Your Doctor Will Listen by Caroline Harding and Barbara Korsch, MD

www.wrongdiagnosis.com/top-100 (WrongDiagnosis.com)

Medical Terminology

The Patient's Guide to Medical Terminology by Charlotte Isler

Medical Terminology: The Basics: Laminate Reference Chart by Corinne B. Linton

www.mlanet.org/resources/medspeak (Medical Library Association's Deciphering Medspeak)

www.medterms.com (Medical dictionary at WebMD's MedicineNet, Inc.)

Fibromyalgia

www.thegroveapproach.com (The Grove Approach)

Cancer

Annals of Surgical Oncology

European Journal of Oncology

www.cancer.net (Cancer.Net [formerly People Living with Cancer], by the American Society of Clinical Oncology)

www.cancer.gov (National Cancer Institute)

https://cissecure.nci.nih.gov/factsheet (National Cancer Institute, organizations that offer services to those with cancer)

www.cancer.org (American Cancer Society)

Insurance

Fight Your Health Insurer and Win: Secrets of the Insurance Warrior, by Laurie Todd; also www.theinsurancewarrior.com

Patient Safety

Josie's Story by Sorrel King

What You Don't Know Can Kill You, by Laura Nathanson, MD

www.hcqualitycommission.gov (President's Advisory Commission on Consumer Protection and Quality in the Health Care Industry)

www.jointcommission.org (Joint Commission)

www.ihi.org (Institute for Healthcare Improvement)

www.facs.org (American College of Surgeons)

Symptom-Matching

medlineplus.gov (U.S. National Library of Medicine and National Institutes of Health)

webapps.jhu.edu/jhuniverse/medicine/diseases (Johns Hopkins Medical Desk Reference)

www.rarediseases.org (National Organization for Rare Disorders)

www.wrongdiagnosis.com (WrongDiagnosis.com)

www.aarp.org and click on the "Health" banner and then the "Symptom Checker" button (AARP)

The Merck Manual of Diagnosis and Therapy

Diagnostic Tests

www.health.harvard.edu/diagnostic-tests (Harvard Health Publications, Harvard Medical School)

Physician Credentials

webapps.ama-assn.org/doctorfinder (American Medical Association)

www.healthgrades.com (HealthGrades)

http://recognition.ncqa.org/index.aspx

www.abms.org (American Board of Medical Specialties)

Hospital Credentials

www.healthgrades.com (HealthGrades)

www.leapfroggroup.org/for_consumers (The Leapfrog Group)

Clinical Trials

clinicaltrials.gov (National Institutes of Health)

www.cancer.gov/clinicaltrials (National Cancer Institute)

Patient Rights and Privacy

www.hhs.gov/ocr/hipaa (U.S. Department of Health and Human Services)

Screening Tests

women.webmd.com (WebMD)

Locator for Reputable Sites

www.nlm.nih.gov/medlineplus/healthywebsurfing.html (U.S. National Library of Medicine and National Institutes of Health)

Patient Name _____   Date ___/___/___

ATTEMPTED TREATMENTS

Treatment	Dosage	Prescribing Physician	Date(s)	Outcome

Patient Name _____   Date ___ / ___ / ___

CURRENT MEDICATIONS (DAILY)

Name of Medication	Dosage	Purpose

Patient Name _____   Date ___ / ___ / ___

CURRENT MEDICATIONS (AS NEEDED)

Name of Medication	Dosage	Purpose

MEDICATIONS ALLERGIES _____

Patient Name _____ Date ___/___/___

SUPPLEMENTS/ALTERNATIVE TREATMENTS

Name of Medication/Treatment	Dosage	Purpose

Patient Name _____   Date ___/___/___

CHRONIC MEDICAL CONDITIONS

Condition	Positive Test Results	Physician	Treatment Status	

Patient Name _____   Date ___/___/___

PAST HOSPITALIZATIONS

Reason for Hospitalization	Admitting Physician	Date	Hospital	Treatment

Patient Name _____ Date ___/___/___

SURGERY HISTORY

Name of Procedure	Name of Surgeon	Date	Hospital	Reason for Surgery

Acknowledgments

I thank God for giving me this incredible journey and for the strength and wisdom to come out on the other side a stronger, more insightful person. Thank you Dad, Karl, and Brian for your love and support as I wrote this book, support that you offered as you were hurting after Mom went to heaven. I know she is proud of you!

To Dr. Wyatt, thank you for your passion for your profession. You have the dedication to which all physicians should aspire. Thank you for sharing your wisdom and vast experience with me. I could not have taken on this gargantuan task without the time, energy, and resources you generously provided.

To my agent, Les Stobbe, thank you for believing in me when I didn't believe in myself. You saw the potential in this endeavor from the very beginning. I couldn't have done it without your faith in me.

To Harvest House Publishers, many thanks for standing by me and for allowing me extra time to complete this book during the most difficult period of my life. I hope I can make you proud.

To Gail Waller, many thanks for your meticulous editing work and for keeping me on my toes while offering a great deal of encouragement and insight into the publishing industry.

To Linda Nathan, President, Logos Word Design, Inc. (www.logosword.com), thanks for your thorough editing work and for guiding me through the book proposal process. I could not have survived my first writer's conference without you!

To Austin Boyd, thank you for providing the catalyst I needed. May God bless you and your selfless ministry to new writers.

To Lightning Strike & Electric Shock Survivors, International and Mainstay Suites, Pigeon Forge, Tennessee, thank you for helping me arrange interviews and conduct vital research.

To the contributors who generously shared your time, knowledge, and expertise during interviews and on questionnaires, your input has made this book the valuable resource it is. Thank you! I have learned so much from each of you. I am forever changed and a better person because of you.

Contributors

Marianne Adams
Steven Alexander

American College of Surgeons, Chicago, IL

Milton Anthony, LLC, motivational speaker and counselor

Ronald Anderson

Sarah Bell, RN, Huntsville, Alabama, hospital

Mark Blanchard, Mark Blanchard's Power Yoga

Charles A. Blevins, OTA, MS, author of *Solving the Workers' Compensation Puzzle*

Daniel Blumenthal, MD, MPH, professor and chair, Community Health and Preventive Medicine, Morehouse School of Medicine

Joseph Brasco, MD, the Center for Colon and Digestive Disease, Huntsville, Alabama

Brooke Braun, Senior Director, Communications and Media Relations, American Academy of Physician Assistants

Phyllis Brown

Ellen Burchfield

James Conway, Senior Vice President, Institute for Healthcare Improvement

Cheri Cowell, author of *Direction: Discernment for the Decisions of Your Life*

Brett Enabnit, RPh, Propst Drugstore, Huntsville, Alabama

Dino Ferrante, MD, the Center for Colon and Digestive Disease, Huntsville, Alabama

Taylor and Grant Getschal

Nancy Greer

Karen Grove, creator of the Grove Approach

Chris Gunter, PhD, Director, Research Affairs, Hudson Alpha Institute for Biotechnology

Brian Hall, CPFT, Washington Sports Club, Chevy Chase, Maryland

Kenneth Hampton, attorney-at-law

Timothy Hawkins

Alan Hedge, PhD, Department of Design and Environmental Analysis, Cornell University School of Medicine

Anthony Houssain, DC, Spine Care LLC, Huntsville, Alabama

Steve Ivey, Manager, Huntsville, Alabama, Recreation Services Department

The Joint Commission, Oakbrook Terrace, Illinois

Joe and Cheryll Jude

Gayla Kidd, Huntsville Assistance Program (Alabama)

Ruth Kriz, MSN, APRN

Rachel Kruspe, MD, the Cancer Center of Huntsville, Alabama

Ivy Larson, CPFT; Andrew Larson, MD, FACS, Medical Director,
    JFK Medical Center Bariatric Wellness and Surgical Institute, and
    authors of *The Gold Coast Cure*

Robert Lesslie, MD, author of *Angels in the ER*

Kathi Limbach, Public Information Specialist, Huntsville-Madison
    County, Alabama, Health Department

Karen Lingar, Director, First Community Senior Select, Huntsville,
    Alabama

Reverends Mark and Leigh Ann Looyenga, Covenant Presbyterian
    Church, Huntsville, Alabama

Lennox Marr, RN, MSN, Nurse Oncology Manager, Huntsville
    Hospital, Alabama

Steve Marshburn, President and Founder, Lightning Strike and Electric
    Shock Survivors, International

Richard C. Mayer, DDS, and staff

Robbin McCord, RN, CHSP, Quality Coordinator/Safety Officer,
    Huntsville Hospital, Alabama

Kathleen Meikus, retired Social Security professional

George C. Morgan, MD, Clinic for Neurology, Huntsville, Alabama

Kristina Moyers

National Cancer Institute, Bethesda, MD

Michael Newman, DVM

The Reverend Hal and Jean Oakley, Covenant Presbyterian Church,
    Huntsville, Alabama

Betty Parcus, CRNP, SPHR, the Boeing Company

Mike Pearce, Minister of Missions, First Baptist Church of Huntsville,
    Alabama

Kevin Ready, ATC, Program Manager, Huntsville Hospital Wellness
    Center, Alabama

J. Thomas Sandy, PhD, Summit Psychotherapy, Huntsville, Alabama

Nancy Schmidt, RN, BSN, Huntsville-Madison County Senior Center, Inc., Alabama

Scott Shapiro, Senior Vice President of Corporate Communications and Marketing, HealthGrades

J. Ellis Sparks, MD, medical library, UAB School of Medicine, Huntsville, Alabama, Campus

Denise Stafford

The faculty physicians of the West Virginia University School of Medicine

Laurie Todd, author of *Fight Your Health Insurer and Win: Secrets of the Insurance Warrior*

Dan Tripp, owner of Head-to-Toe Training, Madison, Alabama

Celia Lloyd-Turney, MD, Director, Choice Medicine, Toney, Alabama

Erin Waddell, Patient Advocate, Fairmont General Hospital, Fairmont, West Virgina

Phillip C. Watkins, MD, Director, the Autonomic Disorders and Mitral Valve Prolapse Center, Birmingham, Alabama

West Virginia University Hospitals

Linda and Wes Whitley and Mitchell Tate

Martha Whitney, MH, HOM, Health in Hand, Eva, Alabama

Sandra J. Williams

Madison County Department of Human Resources, Huntsville, Alabama

Lawrence Wilson, Senior Pastor, Fall Creek Wesleyan Church, Fishers, Indiana, and author of *Why Me? Straight Talk about Suffering*

Terry Wingo, RPh, Madison Drugs, Madison, Alabama

Claire Wood, RN, BSN, Huntsville-Madison County Senior Center, Inc., Alabama

Guide to Medical
Terminology in This Book

Adrenal glands. A pair of endocrine organs that produce the necessary hormones for epinephrine and norepinephrine.

Adrenoleukodystrophy. A rare inherited disease of the central nervous system that causes deterioration of the myelin sheath and affects mostly males in childhood.

Allopathic medicine. Traditional medicine system aimed at combating disease with remedies such as medication or surgery.

Alternative medicine. Healing or disease treatment system not taught in traditional medicine curriculum. Includes homeopathy, naturopathy, acupuncture.

Aneurysm. An abnormal blood vessel dilation filled with blood, often caused by disease of the vessel wall.

Ankylosing spondylitis. Rheumatoid arthritis affecting the spine.

Anorexia nervosa. Eating disorder that typically presents in young women. Characterized by a pathological fear of weight gain, resulting in excessive weight loss and malnutrition.

Arthroscopic surgery. Minimally invasive surgical procedure that uses a small lighted instrument to correct orthopedic and other conditions.

Autonomic nervous system. Consists of the sympathetic and parasympathetic nervous system and governs involuntary action such as secretion and blood pressure.

Bartonella. Gram-negative bacteria, also known as cat scratch disease.

Bisphosphonate. Family of medications used to treat osteoporosis.

Bulimia. A serious eating disorder that results in overeating, followed by self-induced vomiting or laxative abuse.

Carcinoid. A benign or malignant tumor, often from the mucosa of the gastrointestinal tract.

Cardiovascular syncope. Loss of consciousness attributed to abnormality in the cardiovascular system.

Celiac disease. A chronic hereditary disorder in which gluten is not absorbed properly, resulting in an immune response that damages the intestinal mucosa.

Chiari malformation. A congenital abnormality in which the cerebellum and medulla oblongata protrude down into the cervical spinal canal through the opening in the skull.

Colectomy. Surgical removal of all or part of the colon.

Colonoscopy. Examination of the colon using a flexible endoscope.

Connective tissue disease. A disease characterized by inflammation or degeneration of the connective tissue, such as lupus or rheumatoid arthritis.

Conversion disorder. A psychiatric condition in which symptoms appear without a physical explanation.

Crohn's disease. Chronic ileitis that often spreads to the colon, causing diarrhea, bleeding, and malabsorption of nutrients.

CT scan. A scan of the body using computed tomography.

Demyelinating brain disease. Brain disease characterized by the loss or destruction of myelin.

EEG. Electroencephalogram, a test that traces brain waves.

Endoscopy. A test using an illuminated tubular instrument to view the inside of a hollow organ, usually the esophagus.

Ergonomics. Science that studies human characteristics for better designs to help people and things work more safely and efficiently together.

Etiology. Cause of a disease or abnormal physical condition.

Fecal occult. A screening test that checks for blood in the stool.

Gastroenterologist. A specialist who diagnoses and treats conditions of the gastrointestinal tract, the stomach and intestines.

Holistic medicine. A term used to describe therapies that treat the patient as a whole person by looking at that individual's overall physical, mental, spiritual, and emotional well-being before recommending treatment.

Homeopathy. A method of treating a disease using minute doses of a remedy that would result in symptoms of that disease in a healthy person.

Hydronephrosis. Distention of the kidney, caused by an obstruction that forces accumulation of urine into the renal pelvis, causing atrophy of the kidney.

Hypochondriasis. Abnormal level of concern for one's health, often accompanied by delusions of physical symptoms.

Huntington's disease. An inherited disease that often begins in middle age, characterized by mental deterioration and leading to dementia and spasmodic movements of the limbs.

Malingering. The act of exaggerating illness or injury to avoid work or other responsibility.

Medigap. Supplemental insurance plan that covers costs not paid by Medicare.

Metastasis. Spread of disease, such as cancer, from primary site to other areas of the body.

MRI. Magnetic resonance imaging, a noninvasive technique that produces computerized images of internal body tissues based on nuclear magnetic resonance within the body.

MAOI. Monoamine oxidase inhibitor, antidepressant medications that inhibit monoamine oxidase by increasing the level of monoamines in the brain.

Myoclonic jerks. A seizure disorder that consists of a jerking motion of most muscles in the body.

Naturopathy. Treatment of disease that avoids medications and surgery and emphasizes the use of natural agents.

Nephrostomy. Surgical procedure that creates an opening between a renal pelvis and the outside of the body.

Neuropsychiatry. A branch of medicine that combines neurology and psychiatry.

Neuropsychology. A science that integrates psychological observations of behavior and neurological observations of the brain and nervous system.

Opthaneurology. Medical subspecialty that combines the specialties of neurology and ophthalmology.

Orthostatic hypotension. An abnormal decrease in blood pressure when a person stands up; can cause fainting.

Palliative care. An approach to health care that focuses on attending to physical and emotional comfort of patients rather than a cure.

Pathology. The anatomic and physiological abnormalities that indicate the presence of disease or characterize a particular disease.

Peer-reviewed articles. Scholarly articles written by medical professionals that appear in academic journals and are reviewed by medical peers.

PET scan. A view of a particular area of the body, constructed by positron-emission tomography.

Photonic stimulation. Alternative healing protocol that uses infrared light therapy.

Pituitary glands. Gland at the base of the brain that secretes hormones that affect skeletal growth, development of the sex glands, and other functions of the body.

Proprioceptive system. System that regulates the awareness of the body in space.

Pseudo-seizures. Term formerly used to describe psychogenic nonepileptic seizures, a form of conversion disorder.

Psychotherapist. An individual who practices psychotherapy as a clinical psychologist, psychiatrist, or social worker.

Sensory integration dysfunction. A neurological disorder that causes difficulties with processing information from the five senses (vision, hearing, touch, smell, and taste), the sense of movement (vestibular system), or the positional sense (proprioception).

Somatoform condition. Physical ailment such as pain or nausea, or concerns for which no adequate medical explanation has been found.

Stent. A metal or plastic tube, often in the form of a mesh, that is inserted into an anatomical vessel such as an artery or organ to open a previously blocked passageway; also a mold used to keep a surgical graft in place.

Temporal lobes. Part of the cerebrum; involved in auditory processing, semantics both in speech and vision, and memory formation.

Thermography. A technique for detecting and measuring variations in the heat emitted by various areas of the body and transforming them into visible signals that can be recorded photographically.

Thymus. Gland where T cells develop; functions in cell-mediated immunity.

Tilt-table test. Diagnostic medical procedure, often used to diagnose dysautonomia or syncope (fainting).

Tinnitus. A symptom, rather than a disease, that causes ringing, buzzing, whistling, humming, or hissing in the ears.

Triage. The sorting of patients based on the urgency of their need for care in an emergency medical setting.

Ulcerative colitis. A chronic inflammatory disease of the colon characterized by diarrhea with discharge of mucus and blood, cramping abdominal pain, and non-intestinal symptoms such as joint pain.

Ureters. Paired ducts that carry urine away from a kidney to the bladder and open into the pelvis of a kidney and the back part of the bladder.

URL. Uniform resources locator, commonly known as a Web-site address.

Urostomy. An ostomy (appliance that provides artificial elimination) that diverts urine from the body.

Vestibular system. The vestibule of the inner ear, combined with the end organs and nerve fibers that function in mediating the sense of balance.

Sources for the definitions:
www.nlm.nih.gov/medlineplus/mplusdictionary.html
http://medical-dictionary.thefreedictionary.com/

References

Agrawal, A., MD, and Wy Wu, MD. 2009. Reducing medication errors and improving systems reliability using an electronic medication reconciliation system. *Jt Comm J Qual Patient Saf* 35:2 (February): 106–14 <www.ncbi.nlm.nih.gov/pubmed/19241731>.

American Academy of Emergency Medicine. 2009. EMTALA. 22 March 2009 <www.aaem.org/emtala>.

Bell, Chaim M., MD, and Donald A. Redelmeier, MD. 2001. Mortality among patients admitted to hospitals on weekends as compared with weekdays. *New England Journal of Medicine* 345 (August 30): 663–68.

Belling, Barbara. 2004. What is managed care? Office of the Commissioner of Insurance [Wisconsin]. 16 March 2009 <oci.wi.gov/articles/0101mgcr.htm>.

Blevins, Charles A., OTA, MS, and Daniel C. Valdez, MD. 2007. *Solving the Workers' Compensation Puzzle.* Salt Lake City: Aardvark.

Burton, C.V. 2009. Paul Ellwood and the genesis of managed health-care. The Burton Report. 16 March 2009 <www.burtonreport.com/InfHealthCare/ManagedEllwood.htm>.

CMS issues three national coverage determinations to protect patients from preventable surgical errors. 2009. Centers for Medicare and Medicaid Services. 15 January. 30 March 2009 <www.cms.hhs.gov/apps/media/press/release.asp?Counter=3408&intNumPerPage=10&checkDate=&checkKey=&srchType=1&numDays=3500&srchOpt=0&srchData=&keywordType=All&chkNewsType=1%2C+2%2C+3%2C+4%2C+5&intPage=&showAll=&pYear=&year=&desc=&cboOrder=date>.

Cowell, Cheri. *Direction: Discernment for the Decisions of Your Life.* Kansas City: Beacon Hill, 2007.

Cutler, Nicole, Lac. 2006. Effective pain management techniques. Institute for Integrative Healthcare Studies. 16 August. 22 March 2009 <www.integrative -healthcare.org/mt/archives/2006/08/effective_techn.html>.

Gawande, Atul, MD, MPH, et al. 2009. A surgical safety checklist to reduce morbidity and mortality in a global population. *New England Journal of Medicine* 360 (January 29): 491–499 <http://content.nejm.org/cgi/content/ short/360/5/491>.

Goodin, Douglas S., MD. 2009. The causal cascade to multiple sclerosis. *PubMed*, 4 (2) (26 February): e4565 <www.ncbi.nlm.nih.gov/sites/entrez>.

Groopman, Jerome, MD. 2007. *How Doctors Think.* Boston: Houghton Mifflin.

Harding, Caroline, and Barbara Korsch, MD. 1998. *The Intelligent Patient's Guide to the Doctor-Patient Relationship: Learning How to Talk So Your Doctor Will Listen.* New York: Oxford University Press.

Heffernan, Timothy P., PhD, et al. 2009. ATR–Chk1 pathway inhibition promotes apoptosis after UV treatment in primary human keratinocytes: potential basis for the UV protective effects of caffeine. *Journal of Investigative Dermatology* 26 February. 19 March 2009 <www.nature.com/search/ executeSearch?sp-q-9=JID&sp-q=heffernan&sp-x-9=cat&sp-a=spl001702d&sp -sfvl-field=subject%7Cujournal&sp-x-1=ujournal&sp-p-1=phrase&sp -p=all&submit=go> doi: 10.1038/jid.2008.435.

Helm, Standiford II, MD. 2009. Pain management. MedicineNet.com. 21 Mar 2009 <www.medicinenet.com/pain_management/article.htm>.

Herzlinger: Announcing new book. 2007. Manhattan Institute for Policy Research. 31 March 2009 <www.manhattan-institute.org/healthcare>.

Holick, Michael F., MD, PhD. 2007. Vitamin D deficiency. *New England Journal of Medicine* 357 (19 July): 266-281.

Hu, Frank B., MD, et al. 2001. Diet, lifestyle and the risk of type II diabetes mellitus in women. *New England Journal of Medicine* 345:790-797.

Information about PAs and the PA profession. 2009. American Academy of Physician Assistants. 22 Mar 2009 <www.aapa.org/geninfo1.html>.

Improving Diagnostic Accuracy, Joint Commission Perspectives on Patient Safety. 7 April 2007 <www.jcrinc.com>.

Klitzman, Robert, MD. 2008. Second opinions, through a patient's eyes. *New York Times,* 12 February. 19 March 2009 <www.nytimes.com/2008/02/12/health/ views/12essa.html>.

Kohn, L.T., J.M. Corrigan, and M.S. Donaldson, eds. 1999. *To Err is Human: Building a Safer Health System.* Institute of Medicine, Committee on Quality of Health Care in America. Washington, DC: National Academies Press.

Lafata, Jennifer Elston, PhD. 2004. False positive cancer screening tests result not only in anxiety but also additional economic costs. *Medical Research News.* 14 December. 18 March 2009 <www.news-medical.net/?id=6856>.

Lagasse, Robert S., MD. 2002. Anesthesia safety: model or myth? a review of the published literature and analysis of current original data. *Anesthesiology* 97:6 (December): 1609-17.

Leape, L., et al. 1991. The nature of adverse events in hospitalized patients. Results of the Harvard Medical practice study II. *New England Journal of Medicine* 324 (February 7): 377–384.

Managing chronic pain: choosing a multidisciplinary pain program. 2009. American Chronic Pain Association. 19 March. 22 March 2009 <www.theacpa.org/people/pain_program.asp>.

Meek, Will, PhD. 2007. Five stages of grief. Psych Central. 24 Feb. 30 March 2009 <psychcentral.com/blog/archives/2007/02/24/five-stages-of-grief>.

Meyer, Joyce. 2005. *Approval Addiction.* New York: Warner Faith.

Miserandino, Christine. 2003. The spoon theory. But You Don't Look Sick. 22 March 2009 <www.butyoudontlooksick.com/the_spoon_theory>.

Moore, Tim. 2009. General Worker's Comp Tips and Worker's Compensation Advice to Avoid Problems on Claims. www.DisabiltySecrets.com. 30 March 2009 <www.disabilitysecrets.com/workers-comp-workmans-compensation-tips.html>.

Nathanson, Laura, MD. 2007. *What You Don't Know Can Kill You: A Physician's Radical Guide to Conquering the Obstacles to Excellent Medical Care.* New York: HarperCollins.

Niebuhr, Reinhold. 1943. "Serenity Prayer." AllAboutGod.com. 22 March 2009 <www.allaboutprayer.org/serenity-prayer.htm>.

Office of Legislative Policy and Analysis. 2009. Legislative Updates. 23 March. 23 March 2009 <olpa.od.nih.gov/legislation/107/pendinglegislation/4access.asp>.

Oz, Mehmet, MD, and Michael Roizen, MD. 2006. *You: The Smart Patient: An Insider's Handbook for Getting the Best Treatment.* New York: Free Press.

Prater, Erin. 2008. Chronic illness in marriage. Focus on the Family. 22 March 2009 <www.focusonthefamily.com/marriage/facing_crisis/chronic_illness.aspx>.

Preidt, Robert. 2009. Wine may be protective against esophageal cancer. Medline Plus. US National Library of Medicine and the National Institutes of Health. 2 March. 30 March 2009 <www.nlm.nih.gov/medlineplus/news/full story_81191.html>.

President's Advisory Commission on Consumer Protection and Quality in the Health Care Industry. 1998. Appendix A Consumer Bill of Rights and Responsibilities. 17 Jul. 30 March 2009 <www.hcqualitycommission.gov/final/append_a .html#chpt8>.

Reason: PS 101, Fundamentals of Patient Safety; Lesson 4: Error versus harm. Institute for Healthcare Improvement. IHI Open School. 31 March 2009 <courses .ihi.org/lesson_view/18/I/index3>.

Rector-Page, Linda, ND, PhD. 1992. *Healthy Healing: An Alternative Healing Reference.* Healthy Healing Publications.

Rubin, Jordan S., NMD, CNC. 2002. *Patient, Heal Thyself: A Remarkable Health Program Combining Ancient Wisdom with Groundbreaking Clinical Research.* Topanga, CA: Freedom Press.

Siva, Nayanah 2005. "Positive effects with Lorenzo's Oil." *The Lancet Neurology* 4 no. 9 (September): 529.

United States of America page. 2009. World Health Organization. 16 March 2009 <www.who.int/countries/usa/en>.

Warren, Rick. 2002. *The Purpose-Driven Life.* Grand Rapids, MI: Zondervan.

Why not the best? Results from the national scorecard on U.S. health system performance, 2008. The Commonwealth Fund. July 17. 16 Mar 2009 <www .commonwealthfund.org/Content/Publications/Fund-Reports/2008/Jul/Why -Not-the-Best--Results-from-the-National-Scorecard-on-U-S--Health-System -Performance--2008.aspx>.

Wilson, Lawrence W. 2005. *Why Me? Straight Talk about Suffering.* Kansas City: Beacon Hill Press.

Wysowski, Diane K., PhD. 2009. Reports of esophageal cancer with oral bisphosphonate use. *New England Journal of Medicine* 360:89-90.

Zaidi, Amir, MRCP, et al. 2000. Misdiagnosis of epilepsy: many seizure-like attacks have a cardiovascular cause. *Journal of the American College of Cardiology* 36, no. 1 (July): 181.

Index

About the Authors

Lisa Hall is a passionate patient advocate as a result of her nearly ten-year search for the correct diagnosis and treatment of a mysterious debilitating medical condition. She has a BS degree in industrial psychology from Fairmont State College and an MS degree in industrial relations from West Virginia University. Upon graduation, she worked for nine years as a human resources administrator for a large aerospace company.

Lisa has published her writing in a collection of lightning survivor stories entitled *Life After Shock: 49 LS&ESSI Members Tell Their Story* (Morris Publishing: 2000), and she also wrote a chapter in the book *Reasonable Accommodations: Profitable Compliance with the Americans with Disabilities Act* (St. Lucie Press: 1996). She was the subject of a *Health* magazine article in 2001.

Because of her newfound passion for patient safety and quality care, Lisa now works in medical marketing in Alabama and is starting her next book in the health-care genre.

Ronald Wyatt, MD, MHA, is a dedicated primary-care physician with 21 years' experience in a clinical practice. He is a 1985 graduate of the University of Alabama School of Medicine, Birmingham, and completed his residency in internal medicine at the University of St. Louis School of Medicine in 1988.

Dr. Wyatt's passion for patient-centered care is not limited to his clinical practice. He previously served as medical director of a community clinic and Chair of Utilization Review at a medical center. He earned an MS degree in health administration from the University of Alabama in Birmingham in 2007. He recently completed the clinical effectiveness program at the Harvard School of Public Health and the Harvard Medical School, with a concentration in health policy, quality improvement, clinical epidemiology, and clinical biostatistics.

Dr. Wyatt is currently a George C. Merck Fellow at the Institute for Healthcare Improvement for 2009–2010 and a practicing internist at the Huntsville Hospital Madison Internal Medicine Clinic in Madison, Alabama.

The Proactive Patient Web Site

For additional resources, please visit **www.theproactivepatient.com**. You will find all the forms recommended in chapter 4 of this book available for download.

The blog on the Web site will help you stay up to date on timely medical topics. You will also find links to helpful sites with information on healthy living, medical research, physician–patient relationships, misdiagnosis, alternative health care, and medical-insurance issues.

Other Harvest House resources to help you
feel better, look better, and live healthy

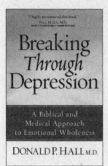

Breaking Through Depression
A Biblical and Medical Approach to Emotional Wholeness
Donald P. Hall, MD

> *"I highly recommend this book."*
> —Dr. Paul Meier, founder of the Meier Clinics

Depression has physical, mental, and spiritual consequences. That's why it can be so difficult for you or someone you love to experience renewal. In a balanced, sympathetic approach that comes from years of listening and helping, psychiatrist Donald Hall integrates medical, psychological, and spiritual knowledge to show you how to move from depression to recovery and healing.

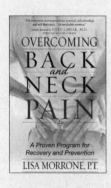

Overcoming Back and Neck Pain
A Proven Program for Recovery and Prevention
Lisa Morrone, PT

From 20 years of teaching and practicing physical therapy, Lisa Morrone gives you a way to say *no* to the treadmill of prescriptions, endless treatments, and a limited lifestyle. This straightforward, clinically proven approach shows you how to strengthen and stretch key muscles, shift to healthy movement patterns, recover from pain caused by injured discs, and address "inside issues" that affect healing.

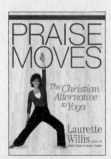

PraiseMoves™
The Christian Alternative to Yoga
Laurette Willis, CPT

Would you like to increase your flexibility, improve your circulation, and enhance your level of energy? *PraiseMoves* offers proven stretching and flexibility exercises without troubling Eastern influences. Now you can fill your mind with Scripture as you promote your health, relieve stress, and grow in God. Transform your workouts into worship with *PraiseMoves!*

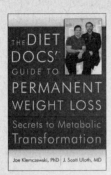

The Diet Docs'® Guide to Permanent Weight Loss
Secrets to Metabolic Transformation
Joe Klemczewski, MD, and J. Scott Uloth, MD

Drs. Scott Uloth and Joe Klemczewski help you put an end to yo-yo dieting by giving you what you need most: control! This is the last diet book anyone will need...written by a family physician partnered by a professional bodybuilder and nutritionist to the world's top bodybuilders and women's figure competitors.

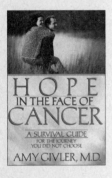

Hope in the Face of Cancer
A Survival Guide for the Journey You Did Not Choose
Amy Givler, MD

Starting from the affirmation that cancer is a treatable disease, Dr. Amy Givler, a cancer survivor herself, gives you solid medical and spiritual guidance—along with personal stories and examples—that will make it easier to deal with decisions about treatment, interact with doctors and hospitals, and understand that spiritual questions are not only normal, but can be welcomed.

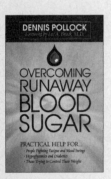

Overcoming Runaway Blood Sugar
Practical Help for: People Fighting Fatigue and Mood Swings • Hypoglycemics and Diabetics • Those Trying to Control Their Weight
Dennis Pollock

With this positive, can-do approach, you can gain maximum health while losing excess pounds. You'll discover why runaway blood sugar is a key factor in food cravings and weight issues, how blood-sugar problems lead to damage to your body, ways to evaluate pre-diabetes health risks, and diet and exercise that really work.

To learn more about other Harvest House books
or to read sample chapters, log on to our website:

www.harvesthousepublishers.com

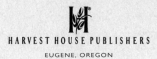

HARVEST HOUSE PUBLISHERS
EUGENE, OREGON